'This regime is easy to stick to because it not only makes perfect sense but it works. You feel better, you look better, you are better.'

Sally Burton

'In 1986, traditional medicine tried for six months – and failed – to sort out the after-effects of salmonella. Gudrun helped me to heal within a fortnight, as well as teaching me to strengthen my immune system and maintain a healthy metabolism.'

Nickolas Grace

'I shall be eternally grateful to Nickolas Grace who gave me his appointment with Gudrun when I was in a state of crisis in my personal and professional life. Gudrun pulled me back to "normal" with amazing speed and I always look forward to my regular maintenance visits.'

Sîan Philips

'Gudrun, you are the best plumber I know!'

Alex Kingston

'Eating is human but digestion is divine.'

(Iranian saying)

GUT REACTION

A revolutionary programme that kick-starts your digestion and detoxes your body system

Gudrun Jonsson
with Tessa Rose

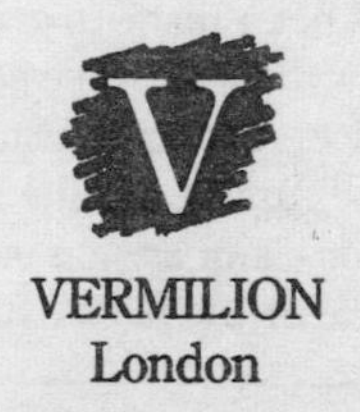

VERMILION
London

7 9 10 8

First published in the United Kingdom in 1998 by Vermilion

This new edition first published in 1999 by Vermilion
an imprint of Ebury Press
Random House
20 Vauxhall Bridge Road
London SW1V 2SA

Random House Australia (Pty) Limited
20 Alfred Street, Milsons Point, Sydney,
New South Wales 2061, Australia

Random House New Zealand Limited
18 Poland Road, Glenfield,
Auckland 10, New Zealand

Random House (Pty) Limited
Endulini, 5A Jubilee Road,
Parktown 1292, South Africa

The Random House Group Limited Reg. No. 954009

www.randomhouse.co.uk

A CIP catalogue record for this book is available from the British Library

ISBN: 0 09 181678 5

Printed and bound in Great Britain by
The Guernsey Press Co. Ltd., Guernsey, Channel Islands

In love and gratitude to the three 'mothers' in my life:

Nan Beecham Moore, who made me understand the links between well-being and upbringing.

Yvonne Trubere, who opened my eyes to the spiritual dimension and the value of leaving a trail of light.

Kate Lomax, who taught me how the 'puzzle' works and sees a glimmer of hope in every situation.

To my village in Sweden, which gave me the freedom of being me without fear throughout my childhood.

CONTENTS

Preface 9

What is a Healthy Person? 11

Chapter One: Understanding the Gut 13

Chapter Two: Pathways to Awareness 27
- The Route to Perfect Digestion 27
- Diet 32
- Exercise 38
- Medication 39
- Stress 40

Chapter Three: Pathways to Regeneration 43
- The Nature of Illness 43
- Restoring the Balance 49
- Change 63

Chapter Four: Treatment Programmes 69
- Asthma 70
- Catarrh/Sinusitis 73
- Constipation 75
- Cystitis 78
- Food Poisoning 79
- Gout 81
- Haemorrhoids 82
- Headache 84
- High Blood Pressure 86
- High Cholesterol 89
- Impotence 91
- Indigestion 94
- Insomnia 95
- Irritable Bowel Syndrome 96
- Joint Problems 100
- Low Blood Sugar 102
- ME 108
- Migraine 111
- Panic Attacks 114
- PMS 116
- Skin Disorders 117
- Ulcer 120
- No Frills Option 123

Chapter Five: Foods, Supplements and Remedies 124

Appendix: Techniques and Recipes 146

The pH Test 146
Boosting the Immune System 147
Refreshing the System 149
Whole Lemon and Olive Oil Drink 151

Acknowledgements, Resources and Further Reading 152

Index 155

PREFACE

This book is about making your health and life simpler to manage. Health can be a complicated business, but my experience as a practitioner in the field has taught me that it need not be.

When I started out as a therapist I quickly became bound up in the minutiae of prescribing vitamins, minerals and all kinds of remedies. Eventually I realized that I was losing sight of the fundamentals of health, such as diet, lifestyle, temperament, genetic blueprint. Good or better health does not come ready labelled in a bottle. To my way of thinking it is a distillation of our real selves, and it can be distilled by us to an easy recipe.

I want to show you how to become sensitive to who you are and what physical, emotional and spiritual needs you can cope with. If you find you cannot cope, I will show you what sort of help you need to ensure that you can cope in future.

We need take only a few gentle steps to change our lives for the better. Solutions can be simple and yet effective. I want to share these solutions with you.

WHAT IS A HEALTHY PERSON?

In clinical terms a healthy person is one in whom disease is not detectable. The majority of us would fit this description. When someone is found to have something wrong with them they will often be said to have been 'struck down by an illness'. The tendency is to dissociate ourselves from the problem, as though it flew in through the window uninvited. To a large extent, however, we make our own health bed, and the minor ailment afflicting us today is a warning sign that worse is almost certainly lurking round the corner if we do not take steps to avoid it. Health is a continuum.

To me a healthy person is like a child: bright-eyed, busy, looking forward to what each day will bring. Many adults get up each morning with that sinking feeling of 'Oh God, I've got to go to work' or 'I wish I didn't have to do that'. When we are healthy, it is as though the sun is always shining, even on rainy days. Life in general, too, seems to run more smoothly and we are able to take any difficulties that arise in our stride. So, how can this Nirvana be achieved?

The answer lies in an area of our anatomy that is often completely overlooked: the digestive system. My work has shown me that the seeds of illness are sown in faulty digestion. When I was training to be a biopath* I was taught that illness could be turned around by the use of vitamins and minerals. Most of my colleagues belonged to one faction or another: one group would push Vitamin E as a cure-all, another Vitamin C, and so on. The more I studied the greater became my conviction that a barrowload of any vitamin will count for nothing if the body is unable to absorb it because of poor digestion. Malabsorption sounds like something that occurs only when someone is very ill or elderly. Unfortunately, it is happening to most of us most of the time, even to those who pride themselves on buying only high quality meat, fish, fruit, vegetables and wholefoods. In addition, these same foods are

* Biopathy was founded by Danish author and therapist Kurt Nielsen and is based on the German system of complex homeopathy.

building up in the digestive system as toxins, undermining our vitality, our immunity to disease and ultimately our health. Very few people realize that *how* we eat has as much effect on the body as *what* we eat.

I have been trying to get this message across to the people who come to my practice. Whatever problem a patient brings to me, we start by working on the digestion and putting that right before considering any additional form of treatment. A poorly functioning digestive system is like a polluted garden pond. Poisoning leads to stagnation and the gradual death of the organisms on which the whole system relies. If toxicity continues to build up in our system, eventually it will incapacitate us through serious diseases such as arthritis, heart disease and cancer. If we could learn to look after the digestive system as diligently as we do other parts of the body, we would be well on the way to curing many of the industrialized world's major diseases.

The principal aim of this book is to show how healthiness can be attained by reducing toxicity in the body, and then maintained by keeping the body free of impurities. For reasons that will become obvious as you read the book, not just the body benefits from cleansing. A clear system has a wonderfully beneficial effect on the mind, the emotions and the spirit. When the digestive system is working efficiently and is not over-loaded, we become aware of ourselves in a totally new way. Suddenly, we have more energy at our command, and we are stronger than any external irritation or problem confronting us. We are quiet, calm and confident. We are clear-headed. Concentration comes easily because our body is uncluttered by debris. If this book has a gift to bestow, it is the knowledge that by taking a few simple measures we can feel so much better about ourselves in all respects, and fulfil our potential as human beings.

Chapter One

UNDERSTANDING THE GUT

The digestion forms the basis of our immune system, and if we want to be healthy – and stay that way – we must make sure our digestion is sound. It is a common misconception to identify the immune system as the white blood cells (leukocytes) that defend the body against invading organisms. In truth the immune system has no separate identity – it is the totality of our organs and tissues working synergistically. How well it functions is a measure of our internal strength. In this chapter we will be looking at how the digestive system is meant to work and the principal reasons why it so often does not.

The Weak Link

The gut is potentially the weakest point in the body. Skin has layers of cells to protect it against toxins. Most organs, like the lungs and the liver, have an enormous capacity to be over-worked. The gut has only one layer of protection.

Given its vulnerability, which is essentially ours too, it is ironic that this should be the most under-valued and abused part of our anatomy, our own Cinderella. In the case of the gut, out of sight really is out of mind – breasts, buttocks and biceps are far more alluring to the imagination and pleasing to the eye than a maze of slimy, palpitating piping. Its workings are about as interesting to the majority of us as the average low-flush cistern. If the ball-cock plays up in the cistern, we call a plumber or tinker with it ourselves. If we have indigestion, we go to the doctor or take an antacid tablet. Life goes on.

With the gut we know that if we put something in at one end, eventually out it will pop at the other. Sometimes we will be aware of how eventful that journey was, sometimes not. Unless we are unfortunate enough to suffer with our digestion or have to watch what we eat, we do not give it a thought until it gives us cause. Usually that cause announces itself in middle age, by which time we have been conditioned into thinking that we cannot expect anything else. Having crested the rise, we are now beginning the descent to decrepitude. We shrug, then have another drink, piece of cake, cigarette or whatever else helps us to forget about ourselves.

Whatever the official name given to the affliction we may be experiencing at this point in our lives, the likelihood is that the gut will have been its port of entry into the system. The fundamental role the gut plays in our emotional and physical well-being is only just beginning to be understood by scientists. The gut, they now realize, has a mind of its own.

The Intelligence Below

Until relatively recently conventional wisdom held that the central nervous system controlled the gut and that the gut itself was merely a tube with simple responses. In fact, the gut has its own brain called the enteric nervous system, which is situated in the sheaths of tissue lining the oesophagus, stomach, small intestine and colon. This brain is composed of 100 million nerve cells (neurons), more than are found in the spinal cord, as well as neurotransmitters and proteins. Almost every chemical substance known to be involved in controlling the brain in the head – including serotonin, two dozen brain proteins (neuropeptides), a class of the body's natural opiates and some psychoactive chemicals – is a component of this enteric nervous system, as are major cells of the immune system.

Through its two networks of nerves (called the myenteric plexus and the submucosal plexus), the brain in the gut controls the rate of digestion, the movement and secretions of the mucous lining the intestines, and the contractions of the various muscles in the gut wall. In this lower brain there are mast cells involved in immune responses, cells that nourish nerve cells and a blood-brain barrier that keeps harmful substances away from important nerve cells. There are also sensors for sugar, protein, acidity and other factors that determine how the gut mixes and moves its contents.

The mucosa of the small intestine is composed of finger-like projections called villi within which reside white blood cells called enterocytes. These are the fastest-growing cells in the body, with renewal occurring every 72 hours. The growth of the enterocytes relies on the presence of digesting food inside the tube (lumen) of the digestive tract. The enterocytes take the nutrients they absorb from digested food to tiny blood vessels inside the villi which lead to the circulatory system by way of the liver. Also residing in the mucosal lining are special white blood cells called lymphocytes, the brains of the immune system, which protect us against anything that should not be there. All of the white cells work together, relaying messages to each other and receiving them from the outside world.

The principal fuel of the mucosal lining is an amino acid called glutamine. This contains two atoms which deposit nitrogen where it is needed in the body and pick it up from where it is not needed; these atoms will, for example, deliver nitrogen to build up muscle or remove it from where there is too much acid, thus helping to keep the body clear of toxins. Glutamine contributes to the production of glutathione peroxidase, one of the body's most important antioxident enzymes and one of the main scavengers against free radicals (see page 25); glutathione is the principal chemical used by the liver, the body's major detoxifying organ.

The brain in the gut will try to deal with whatever we put into our bodies. However, its cells can be deactivated or misfire if they are not properly programmed by us, causing infections to arise from undigested or toxic matter. Malfunctioning within the gut's brain is now thought to be responsible for many gastro-intestinal disorders, including most ulcers, colitis and irritable bowel syndrome, and it may allow life-threatening diseases to develop.

The brain above and the brain below derive from the same clump of tissue called the neural crest, and are connected by the two thousand or so nerve fibres of the vagus nerve. However, the two function independently, and the relationship between them seems to be complementary. The degree to which the enteric nervous system works independently and yet in harmony with its counterpart is startling. Research has shown how the two brains can influence and upset each other. Researchers in the United States estimate that a quarter of the people taking anti-depressants such as Prozac suffer from diarrhoea, constipation or nausea because these drugs act on the serotonin in the gut. Similarly, drugs like morphine and heroin attach to the gut's opiate receptors, causing constipation.

At night the brain in our head sets a pattern of 90-minute cycles of slow wave sleep interspersed with periods of rapid eye movement sleep (when we dream). Meanwhile, as we sleep, the gut's brain produces 90-minute cycles of slow wave muscle contractions interspersed with short bursts of rapid muscle movements. Patients with bowel problems are known to have abnormal rapid eye movement sleep. One explanation for this is that the two brains influence each other during this phase. This idea is not so far-fetched if we recall that certain foods can cause us to have nightmares or bad quality sleep.

Interestingly, the sensations that come from the gut are not all bad. The gut, it is thought, can produce its own feel-good factor, in a series of compounds identical to benzodiazepine, a drug that relieves anxiety.

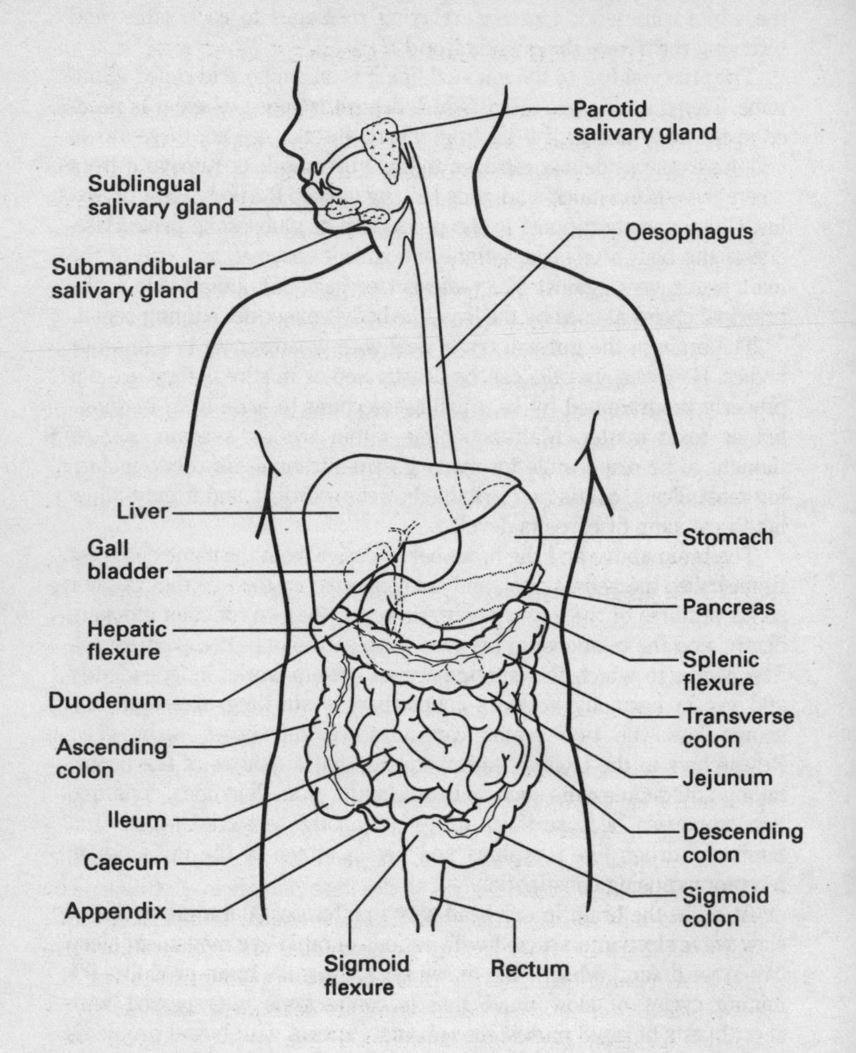

THE DIGESTIVE SYSTEM

Close-up of the Digestive System

One of the least understood facts about the digestive system is the key role it plays in the body's immune system. The skin is the first protective barrier we possess, the second is the intestines, and the third the cells. In effect only the protective buffer offered by the intestines stands between us and illness. Let us take a closer look at the front-line troops of the intestines' defence system.

The surface area of the digestive tract is equal to that of two tennis courts. Gel lines this tract from its starting point, the mouth, to its end, the anus. Everyone knows that between these two points are situated several organs central to the digestive process – for example, stomach, liver and pancreas. Less well known, but critical to an understanding of how the body may remain healthy, are the microflora that live in the gut lining. This biologically active mass has a profound effect on our physiological processes, and is as important to the body as the major organs.

The normal person is composed of over 10^{14} cells. Ninety per cent of these cells are microbial, and most of these live in the gut. In short, the gut holds more bacteria than the human body does cells. There are about 400 to 500 different species of these bacteria or microflora. Some of them have a symbiotic relationship with the body, the gastro-intestinal tract and the mucosa and play a role in metabolizing nutrients, vitamins, drugs, the body's hormones and carcinogens, synthesizing short chain or saturated fatty acids, giving protection against germs and activating the immune system. Others cause disease or are opportunistic. A large quantity of microflora have yet to be classified.

The number of microflora remains more or less stable over time. What can change is the nature of the flora and their condition. The most important species of microflora is *Lactobacillus acidophilus*, which keeps the digestive tract healthy by promoting absorption and digestion, and, vitally, enabling the *Bifido bacterium bifidum* to thrive; the *Bifido bacterium* is the body's army of detoxifiers and defenders against bacterial and viral infection. If this micro-biological state becomes unbalanced, and the number of opportunistic or disease-causing bacteria overwhelms the number of beneficial bacteria, the absorption walls in the small intestine will become ulcerated (what are called 'leaky') and allow toxins to pass into the lymphatic system. Immune deficiencies will result from this process, even if the individual's diet is good.

Before 1979 no known organism could withstand stomach acid. In that year the bacterium *Helicobacter pylori* was discovered. This organism was found to be the causative agent in a vast majority of cases of ulcerated or inflamed stomachs. The bacterium, which grows in the cells of the stomach lining, is protected from stomach acid by an alkaline cloak. Once established in the stomach wall the bacterium releases a cytotoxin that causes cell damage unless the body's immune response is sufficiently robust.

How the Digestion Works

The nature of our digestive problems becomes clearer if we look at how the digestive system works. Put crudely the digestive system is our own personal power plant. It is a common fallacy that the body takes only what it needs and eliminates the rest. If this were true, no one would have bad digestion and far fewer people would develop illnesses. It is more accurate to say that when it is working as it should, it takes what we put in and converts it into energy for us to use for repair or growth. Before considering the problems that commonly arise because of this yawning gap between hope and experience, let us first briefly look at the mechanics of digestion and the roles different parts of the digestive system play in that process.

Mouth

This is where digestion begins, and usually goes wrong (but more of that later). Saliva plays a crucial role in digestion and absorption. As we chew so enzymes are released which begin the process of breaking down fats and starches and messaging the stomach that proteins are on their way.

Stomach

Food is mechnically churned in the stomach and treated with more enzymes. One to two litres (two to three and a half pints) of gastric juices – including hydrochloric acid and miscellaneous enzymes – are secreted by cells in the stomach wall to break down protein molecules, help kill bacteria in food and make some minerals (for example, calcium) and iron more absorbable. The stomach emulsifies fat, and fat globules are dispersed for pancreatic enzymes to split triglycerides into fatty acids and monoglycerides, as well as to break down various polyesters. The gastric enzymes have weak fat-splitting ability.

Small intestine

About 25 mm (1 inch) in diameter and six metres (20 feet) long, the small intestine is made up of the duodenum, the jejenum (Latin for 'empty') and the ileum (from the Greek 'eileos', meaning 'twisted'). It is arranged as folds and projections which, if laid out flat, would cover an area the size of a football pitch. The greater part of digestion and absorption of all nutrients – that is, the products of digestion of dietary carbohydrate, protein and fat, the remains of the digestive juices, and minerals and vitamins – takes place at this point in the system, through enzymes secreted by the pancreas, Crypts of Lieberkuhn, and the liver.

Duodenum

This is the first 300 mm (12 inches) of intestine nearest the stomach and is the entry port through which juices flow into the intestines. The hormone secretin is released as partly digested food enters the duodenum from the stomach. Fat and acid pulp (food converted by gastric secretions) stimulate the production of secretin, which is carried in the blood to the pancreas.

Pancreas

The pancreas secretes juices at the rate of 2.5 litres (4$^1/_2$ pints) per day under the control of the vagus nerve and the duodenal hormone secretin. This alkaline juice neutralizes the acid mixture from the stomach. Among the enzymes contained in this juice are trypsin, amylase and lipase, which act respectively on protein, starch and fat. The pancreas also produces the hormone insulin, which flows into the bloodstream to be used around the body to assist the entry of glucose to cells.

Crypts of Lieberkuhn

Found in the mucosa of the small intestine, these produce small amounts of digestive enzymes and immunoglobins (proteins that act on antibodies).

Liver

This organ secretes 700 ml (1$^1/_4$ pints) of bile each day which is stored in the gall bladder, a sac-like structure about the size of a purse. Bile emulsifies fat, breaking it down into smaller and smaller globules so that it can be chemically split by the pancreatic digestive juices before entry into the bloodstream through the wall of the small intestine. Poisonous substances in the body go directly from the intestines to the liver via the portal vein where they are removed from the blood.

Large intestine

About one and a half metres (5 feet) long and 50 mm (2 inches) in diameter the large intestine is principally the exit route for the body's waste, including toxins. The first part of the large intestine, the ascending colon, is on the right side of the body. The portion crossing the body from left to right is the transverse colon. The portion on the left side of the body, where the waste travels down and out via the anus, is the descending colon. The main role of the large intestine is to absorb about 1 litre (1¾ pints) of water daily to assist the passage of waste.

What the Body Takes

The absorption of individual components from the nutrients we ingest takes place throughout the system – in theory.

Mouth

Very little is absorbed here, but saliva re-mineralizes the teeth with calcium salts.

Stomach

Alcohol, sugar, soluble mineral salts (for example, sodium and potassium), water-soluble vitamins (for example, B group vitamins and Vitamin C) are absorbed here.

Small intestine

Most dietary protein is absorbed in the upper jejenum, in the form of amino acids. These acids enter the bloodstream via the intestinal wall and are then carried to the liver and other tissues, where they are used in a number of chemical reactions, including the synthesis of body proteins, nucleic acids and some hormones. The majority of amino acids are processed for use in the production of energy; in the liver, one of their four components, nitrogen, is removed and eliminated as urea by the kidneys, leaving the other three (carbon, hydrogen and oxygen) to be used as fuel.

Carbohydrates are split into monosaccharides in the small intestine before passing into the blood. Any indigestible cellulose or similar material passes into the large intestine.

Fats are absorbed into the lymph via the intestinal wall and then carried to the bloodstream. They are deposited in depots from which they may be drawn as required by the body, and also used in the liver and muscles for the production of energy.

Soluble salts, calcium, iron, water-soluble vitamins of the B group and Vitamin C, and the fat-soluble vitamins A and D are absorbed in the small intestine.

Liver

Sugars are stored here – and also in the muscles – as glycogen. When the body needs energy the glycogen is converted back into glucose (in which guise it reached the liver) and passed into the blood. Much of the energy used by the muscles and the tissues is derived from free fatty acids in the blood. The liver plays an important role in the metabolism of glutamine (see page 134), which is essential to the process of converting fats and sugars. Glutamine is produced by the liver when the body needs it or adapted when it does not; when it is surplus to requirements glutamine is either converted to other amino acids or to nitrogen, which is excreted as waste in the form of urea.

How the System Can Go Wrong

The first chance the digestion gets to go wrong is in the mouth, with carbohydrates. The saliva in the mouth should be alkaline (see The Balancing Agent, page 24), but in most people it is not alkaline enough, which means the stomach, and then the liver and the pancreas further down the chain have to work harder to secrete enough enzymes to break down the food.

If food is not chewed thoroughly the salivary enzymes, which break down fats (lingual lipase) and convert starch to sugar (salivary amylase), cannot do their job properly before the partly digested matter passes to the stomach. Incomplete chewing will also leave the stomach unprepared for any proteins that might be included in this matter. If the stomach does not receive the message that chewing transmits, gastric acid and pepsin will not be excreted in sufficient quantities and the transformations that have to occur in the duodenum – with the help of alkaline-forming pancreatic enzymes and bile – will not be completed.

The situation is if anything worse with fats, because their digestion and absorption is the most complex part of the whole process. Fat is water insoluble and so the gut has to convert it into a soluble, absorbable form which is then secreted into the lymphatic system.

The end result of this chain of non-communication is malabsorption of the vital nutrients the body needs and a build-up of undigested matter.

Too Little or Too Much Acid?

Gastric acids play a crucial role in digestion and assimilation, particularly of proteins and minerals. They are also principal agents in preventing the overgrowth of bacterial flora in the small intestine. This bacterial overgrowth interferes with the processing of nutrients and the digestion of fat, and reduces the availability of Vitamin B12 for absorption.

What actually happens chemically in the gut turns much conventional wisdom on its head. Too much acid in the stomach is usually blamed for causing indigestion, and yet too little acid is the starting point for this and may be implicated in other health problems. These include asthma, eczema, food allergies, diabetes mellitus, coeliac disease, gastritis, hepatitis, dermatitis, gall-bladder disease, autoimmune disorders, stomach cancer and osteoporosis.

The usual signs of low gastric acidity are:

- Bloating, belching, burning and flatulence just after meals
- A feeling of fullness after eating
- Indigestion, diarrhoea or constipation
- Reactions after eating
- Nausea after taking supplements
- Itchiness around the rectum
- Weak, peeling or cracked fingernails
- Dilated veins in the cheeks and nose (in someone without a drink problem)
- Acne (after adolescence)
- Iron deficiency
- Chronic intestinal infections – eg, parasites, bacteria, yeast
- Undigested food in stools

Undigested matter in the system irritates the gel lining the stomach, stimulating it to produce acid. This response is the digestive system's way of trying to right itself. Fried or sharp food is particularly problematic for a stomach in this condition because the bile – which the system asks the liver to send in order to help it cope – adds to the irritation.

The Alkaline-Acid Equation – Health or Disease

Maldigestion in effect upsets the alkaline/acid balance in the digestive system. If this balance is right, it is chemically impossible for the body to become diseased. However, if conditions are wrong, it becomes chemically impossible for the system to work properly; for example, to absorb iron from meat.

If the acidity in the stomach is right, proteins can be broken down. If it is not, these proteins turn acid and rot into toxic molecules, instead of being digested and then transported to the body tissues. It is through the toxins produced by undigested food that the body becomes poisoned. If the state of the microflora is poor, toxic molecules can burrow through the lining of the gut into the lymphatic system. Once they have entered this channel they can be transported in the lymph to any part of the body.

The greater the degree of degradation of the lining, the more severe the illness. Mouth ulcers are the small 'blossoms' of the fungi, or toxicity, in the digestive system. If the conditions that produced these blossoms remain a constant, serious gastro-intestinal disorders may develop.

A diet high in carbohydrates and protein and low in fibre, lack of physical exercise, stress and medication (especially antibiotics) will encourage an over-growth of microflora, causing an imbalance from which digestive disorders and disease states may arise. An overgrowth in the fungal form of *Candida*, for example, has been implicated by some researchers in cases of food allergy, irritable bowel syndrome, systemic lupus, rheumatoid arthritis, vaginitis, chronic fatigue, PMS-related depression, asthma and indigestion. Such fungi cannot live in an alkaline system.

The Balancing Agent – pH

The vital exchange of energy that should take place when we eat cannot occur if the alkaline/acid balance in the gut is wrong. If the body is working well and the immune system is healthy the acid/alkaline balance in the body regulates itself. This is rarely the case because of the stresses we impose on ourselves, crucially through what we eat and drink. The perfectly functioning human would rarely eat sugar, for example.

pH or 'hydrogen potential' is the measure of how alkaline or how acid we are. This is the most basic control of every aspect of body chemistry, including the hundreds of enzymes that deal with digestion and the assimilation of nutrients. pH is recorded on a scale of 0 to 14 and measures the concentration of hydrogen ions in a solution, in this context saliva or urine. I will show you how to carry out your own self-test of saliva and urine later. First, though, an explanation of what saliva pH can tell us.

A score of 0 on the pH scale means the substance being tested cannot get more acid. At the other end of the scale, 14, the substance cannot get more alkaline. Seven is the median figure – below 7 pH is generally considered acid, above 7 pH alkaline.

The ideal pH number of saliva is 6.4. This indicates balance and equilibrium within the body systems. The pH value of normal saliva rises to 7.2 after we eat in order to help digest carbohydrates, and then drops back. Saliva pH below 6.2 indicates poor absorption of nutrients in the gut and also liver toxicity. Low saliva pH is linked to acid blood, deficiencies in potassium, magnesium, calcium and trace minerals, and a high pulse rate (over 80 beats a minute at rest).

A diet high in refined foods, especially white sugar and grains, is thought to cause acid saliva. Heavy metal poisoning (for example, from pollution), prescription or street drugs, and smoking are also contributory factors.

It is undoubtedly better to have a pH reading that shows you to be just on the alkaline side than just on the acid. However, saliva pH of 6.8 to 7.0 indicates a slow digestion and possibly a shortfall in amino acids and hormones such as thyroxin. The more marked the shift away from 6.4 in either direction, the more serious the imbalance in the body. (See pages 146–147 for saliva/urine test procedures.)

Free Radicals v Antioxidants

The importance of the body being able to absorb sufficient minerals and vitamins becomes clear if we look at the role of so called 'free radicals'. Since the 1980s scientists have become increasingly excited by the decisive influence these rogue electrons have on the development of many diseases. Scientists have linked free radicals to more than 200 illnesses and estimated their damage to account for 70 per cent of all disease, including arteriosclerosis, coronary thrombosis, cerebral haemorrhage, cancer, senility, cataracts and chronic arthritis.

Free radicals are formed out of the chemical reaction which the body undergoes as a result of its exposure to alien substances, such as pollution, radiation, pesticides, food additives, tobacco, alcohol and drugs. The free radical is an unpaired electron (normally electrons are joined in pairs) which then looks to steal an electron from other molecules. During this quest it bombards our cells – imagine meteorites pounding the outer surface of a planet – and these respond by forming enzymes. If a cell is unable to mount a robust defence in the form of the vitamins and minerals that function as antioxidants, and the free radicals break through its shield, disease and ageing are the result. The area of the body where free radicals are most likely to succeed is in the gut where the barrier between toxins and the organs is at its weakest.

Where am I?

In a majority of us the bacterial flora is not in good shape and thus our buffer against disease is compromised as toxins start seeping into the lymphatic. That said, most people are in blissful ignorance of their state and have got into the habit of living with so-called 'minor' ailments. If you answer 'Yes' to just one of the following questions, read on.

1. **Do you feel tired even after a night's sleep?**
2. **Do you find it difficult to relax?**
3. **Do you never have a thirst?**
4. **Are you ravenously hungry before meals?**

5. **Do you experience dips in your energy levels between meals?**
6. **Do you experience a sense of fullness after eating a meal?**
7. **Do you frequently suffer from indigestion, heartburn, burping, wind, constipation or diarrhoea?**
8. **Do you have dry, itchy or greasy skin?**
9. **Do you get headaches?**
10. **Are you overweight?**
11. **Do you often feel gloomy for no apparent reason?**

Few of these questions may seem to hint at a disease state. Indeed, for most of us the question of whether our skin is dry or greasy seems unimportant – we simply buy a moisturizer appropriate to our skin type. If we are tired, we put it down to over-work or too little sleep. If we get hungry between meals we snack on something until the pangs wear off.

A 'Yes' answer to each of the above questions would not strike most people as worth worrying about. And questions 6 and 7 apart, few people would think the topics had anything to do with digestion. In fact, a 'Yes' to any of these questions tells us that the digestion is not working as it should and consequently the microflora are out of balance.

In order to strengthen our buffer, we have to start with the digestion and look at ways of making this work better. Only then will the lymphatic system 'perk up' and gradually be re-energized, correcting imbalances in the body and reducing the possibility of serious disease developing in our organs. When the digestion starts working more efficiently, we begin to feel better both physically and psychologically. We sleep better, we are happier, we cope better – and we can begin to enter 'No' answers to the questions in the list above.

Chapter Two

PATHWAYS TO AWARENESS

Whatever our health problem, the digestion will undoubtedly play a major part in it. The person with the perfect digestive system can eat whatever they like, in whatever combination and not suffer any ill effects. Usually that person is rarely burdened by illness. Conversely, the person with a weak digestive system is burdened by illness, unless they learn to look after themselves in terms of what and how they eat.

We know instinctively what is good for our health, but the boredom quotient in being that sensible is too high for most of us. We prefer to ignore the subtle hints our body at first throws out. We react – usually by taking a stronger pill – only when it starts to make life difficult for us. There is rarely one route to anything, but where the digestion is concerned there are basic, simple rules we should learn. We will look at these before going on to examine each of the four principal minefields that our digestion is forced to cross, under heavy fire, throughout our entire life – diet, exercise, medication and stress

Pathway 1
– THE ROUTE TO PERFECT DIGESTION

The vast majority of us expect to suffer periodic bouts of indigestion, wind, constipation or diarrhoea. These upsets are signs of the gut under pressure, specifically, as we have seen in Chapter One, when at some point in the digestive system the acid/alkaline balance, and thus the microflora, is out of kilter. Someone with perfect digestion goes to the toilet twice a day, never has wind or similar discomfort, never gets a headache, never over-eats, and their level of energy does not fluctuate. The main reason for this state of grace is that they do not overload themselves physically or mentally.

The Crunch Point

Few people fit this description, and even fewer by the time they reach middle age. It is at this point in life when people, who have previously been able to eat any type of food or combination of foods without suffering a twinge of complaint, start to feel and look their age.

Like other parts of the body the digestive system ages and weakens. Depending on strength of constitution and the amount of stress the body has been put under, most people become aware of digestive problems between the ages of 45 and 50. At around this time the body's ability to secrete digestive enzymes reduces by about 40 per cent. There is also a corresponding decrease in the body's ability to absorb nutrients. Middle-age spread is a further reflection of this deterioration in the system's efficiency, and of our failure to compensate for it. We can no longer cope as well with the food we enjoyed formerly. We may feel acidic, be prone to heartburn, or wake up in the middle of the night if we eat too late. Any of these is a sign that we need to re-examine our eating habits, and to lighten the burden we are heaping on our digestive system. It is never too late, even to change the habits of a lifetime. Take heart, as in all things, ageing is relative – the best digestion among all my patients belongs to a spry 78-year-old.

So, how is perfect digestion achieved? The answer is to begin by looking at how we eat and the reasons why so few of us manage to perform adequately the actual mechanics of eating.

Ways of Eating

The way we eat has as much impact on our digestion as what we eat. The most basic cause of the incorrect fermentation that leads to so many of our health problems can easily be put right. Eating only when you are in a calm, relaxed state and chewing each small forkful of food 50 times will produce conditions in the mouth that are absolutely right for digestion. Acid-forming foods can be transformed into alkaline-forming foods by thorough chewing. You will find that some foods – notably grains – become more tasty the longer they are chewed.

- **When you sit down to a meal, think of Mahatma Gandhi's advice to '. . . chew your drinks and drink your foods'.**

This sounds simple enough, but the simple things are invariably the most difficult to do at all, let alone do well. We do not chew our food.

Rarely are we calm. Eating too quickly or while on the move, eating late or skipping meals altogether are all common patterns. To digest a food properly means to ferment it in a very precise manner. If your digestion is poor, and these patterns will make it so, your food cannot be fermented properly and it becomes toxic, even if it is the best food in the world or perfect for other people.

It is up to each of us to find ways of making life more relaxed and less pressured. If we can do that, our digestion will cope better too.

The Headless Chicken Tendency

If you do not sit for a while after a meal but get up immediately and rush off to make the next appointment or complete the next task, you are in effect putting the digestion on hold. The adrenaline that starts pumping as soon as you become active overrides the process of the blood coming to the stomach to assist digestion. Most people with this lifestyle find it very difficult to relax. They have to be induced into letting go. I encourage them to sit with a hot water bottle on the stomach and at the back after meals, so they feel warm and comfortable and the stomach expands. Obviously this can only be done when one is at home. If you have to eat out a lot, perhaps entertaining clients, try to think relaxed and replicate with your mind the good work of that hot water bottle. Use one of life's great health-givers, laughter. When you laugh genuinely, tension evaporates, and your whole digestive system works better.

A GP referred a highly-stressed woman to me whose stomach had blown up like a balloon. She brought her two children with her to the consultation. It became apparent that, whatever I said to her, she would not sit down and eat in a relaxed fashion because she would be too busy organizing everyone else in the family. I asked the children if they would help their Mummy by ensuring that whenever she sat down to eat everyone round the table should tell a funny story. No one should be allowed to leave the table until somebody in the group had made everyone else laugh. The children loved the whole idea of this and it became an enjoyable part of their daily routine. The mother became aware of her own behaviour, of always being up and down and fussing. Gradually she relaxed to the point where she was not concerned if everything was not perfect or she had forgotten something.

One would expect people, who routinely run themselves ragged, to burn up their food and as a result to be as lean as the proverbial rake. The reverse is usually the case, because their food quite literally sits on them and is never properly digested, enlarging throughout the day and resulting in weight gain.

Eating Late

Taking large meals late at night will cause problems with the digestive system. Because the body clock is regulated by the light, digestive enzymes are very reluctant to spring into action after hours, as it were, so whatever we have eaten will tend to sit in our stomachs the whole night long, pressing and ballooning against the heart. In some people this discomfort can make them think they are having a heart attack.

Skipping Meals

If we skip a meal the body will use our adrenaline in compensation for the food it should be getting in order to keep going. Breakfast is typically the meal that many people do without. Instead of taking proper nourishment before setting off for the day, they will artificially energize themselves by drinking a cup of coffee. When we kick-start the body in this way, we are drawing on our nervous energy and draining ourselves. The same applies to the person who does not have lunch. The body will use adrenaline and stress to maintain the correct level of blood sugar. Not surprisingly, the meal-skipping type will tend to be short-tempered and aggressive.

Denying the body proper nourishment at regular intervals throughout the day is a dangerous habit to get into. Anyone who does it is living on borrowed energy, and, if they continue doing it, in the end there will be no energy to take. It is like living on an overdraft facility all the time. One day when you desperately need a bit of extra (when you are ill, for example), you will discover there is no cushion of capital on which to draw.

By eating little and often you will ensure that your digestion copes with whatever you are doing, and that the body is fed as it should be.

Grazing

For people who have low blood sugar (see page 102) or who notice a rapid dip in energy and concentration between meals, it is advisable to eat something every three to four hours. Grazing, or eating a little all the time, is not a good idea, however, because what we are putting in is never properly digested. The body chemistry changes each time we eat, no matter how small the amount – it will change even for a solitary peanut. When the digestion is right we do not need to eat as often and can happily live on three meals a day.

How Much is Too Much?

Some writers dedicated to improving our health suggest that we can eat as much as we like of some foods. They are, perhaps, engaged in a sort of trade-off with the reader – 'I may not allow you to eat this, but you can have unlimited helpings of that'. The greedy element in each of us certainly draws comfort from such encouragement. Unfortunately, volume does matter, even of foods that are very good for us. Several helpings of vegetables is too much at one sitting, no matter how perfectly produced or cooked the vegetables may be.

I can give a wonderful example of a man who went to his summer house and for three weeks ate only lettuce in order to lose weight. The problem was he ate a huge amount of it. His stomach literally blew up and he put on a stone in weight. He could not understand how a food containing virtually zero calories could have had this effect. The point is that his stomach was already fermenting badly and this excess of raw matter was like putting a match to a box of tinder.

By eating more than we need, we distend the gut and make the digestive system work harder than it should. At the end of it we are less healthy because of the toxins arising from that undigested matter. Eating too much makes us tired. Falling asleep in front of the television after we have eaten our evening meal is a sure sign of low energy.

- **As a general rule, at a meal it is best to eat no more than will fill your two hands cupped together. One quarter to a third of the volume should be protein or starch foods and the rest vegetables.**

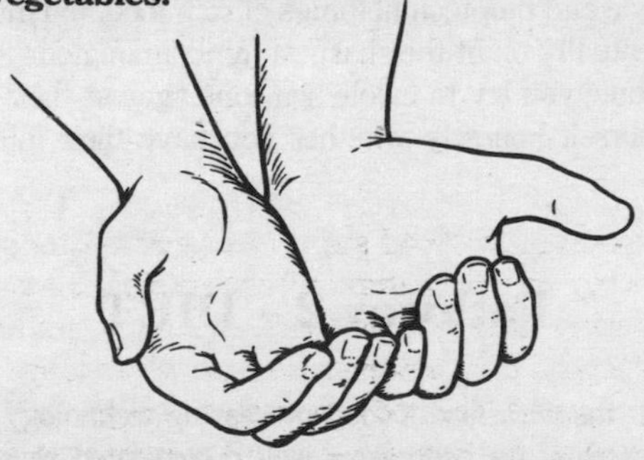

There is also a good practical reason for not eating more. Fresh organic meat, vegetables and fruit are, in my view, better tasting and better for us than processed or refined foods or fresh produce that has been grown with the use of chemicals. They are also more expensive to buy. If someone argues that they cannot afford to buy good food, I reply that if it is eaten in the correct volume, it is affordable. Look at the size of your two hands cupped together – compare it with the amount that you put on your plate. It is far better to eat no more than we need of good food than to eat four times that quantity of low-grade food. Eating less also somehow increases our appreciation of what we do eat. If we cherish that small amount and really savour it, as in so many other areas of life less becomes more.

Whose Comfort Food?

It is interesting how the idea of being allowed to pig ourselves makes us feel comfortable. The person with either perfect digestion, or a well-developed awareness of what is intrinsically good for them, gets a message to stop before crossing the great divide into over-eating. In some social situations it can be difficult to resist the pull across that line. And when we are hosts, more often than not we will contrive to nudge – and sometimes drag – our guests over it.

How many of us are content to let our dinner guests have a little and be happy? The truth is that we want them to get up from the table stuffed. Our cultural training tells us that a good host is a bountiful one – never mind that we are probably shortening our guests' lives by a few years and almost certainly sending them home to a disturbed night of frequent visits to the lavatory or the medicine cabinet. I cannot help wondering if the host wedded to the 'stuff them' principle is not waging a subtle form of social warfare. After the first or second flush of wine-induced sparkle and umpteen helpings of rich food, too much of a good thing will eventually blunt the sharpest mind among our guests.

The next time you try to cajole someone against their better judgement, ask yourself honestly whether you have their interest or your own at heart.

Pathway 2 – DIET

Precisely what the wizardry of food processing technology is costing us in nutritional terms has been very well documented elsewhere. A frequently forgotten aspect of such discussions is the degree to which we in the West have lost sight of the purpose of food. Because so much of it is available, in so many different forms, we tend to treat it as a commodity, like buying a shirt or a ticket to an entertainment. When choosing what we eat the question is not, 'Will it be good for me?' but 'Will it please me?', and because what is good for us is invariably equated with misery or sacrifice, mostly we plump for pleasure. In many cases this attitude translates into a diet consisting of refined carbohydrates and very little else.

Food Wisdom

Food undoubtedly is one of life's great pleasures, but above all it provides nourishment, in the fullest sense of that word. Good food, like good anything, whether it be a piece of music, a painting, a play, a conversation, a relationship, demands something of us. We have to engage with it, experience its essence.

It is very important that food should look and smell wonderful. If it does you are half-way to digesting it well, because your digestive juices will already be flowing richly before you have raised the first forkful to your mouth. Sitting down to eat with other people and generating an atmosphere of conviviality are wonderful stimuli to the digestion too. Good food and serious conversation do not mix. Take time to eat, and then to talk. We are so conditioned to do everything in the shortest possible time that nothing is given its due. Eating is one of the first casualties of the corner-cutting lifestyle. Be serious about what you eat. We should take a leaf out of the average Mediterranean person's book of life – savour our food, talk about it, be interested in it, and never regard it as just another plateful of fuel.

Concentrate on how your food really tastes. Go out of your way to try different vegetables, different herbs, different combinations. If food is tasty, you eat slowly. If it is boring, you eat faster. It is so easy to become set in our ways, to have the same foods week in week out and dismiss the unfamiliar. The first time I had a Japanese meal I thought, 'Gosh, what bland, horrible food'. After a while, though, I came to appreciate the subtlety of the flavours, and now I think the traditional Japanese diet is the best. Much of their food is pre-fermented – their rice and soya, for example – which makes it easier on the digestion. They eat lots of top greens, lightly cooked. Little flour is used in their cooking, and no cow's milk. They are aware, too, of the need to keep the acidity in the gut balanced, and so the meal will invariably include an Umeboshi plum per person, placed on the rice, and fermented pickles.

At some point in our history we too became aware that certain foods needed to be balanced – serving apple with pork and duck or cranberries with turkey or venison are examples of that awareness. We need to re-acquaint ourselves with these old ground rules and develop a few more as far as our digestion is concerned.

Which Foods?

Numerous researches over the years have told us that the average Western diet is high in animal proteins, saturated fatty acids and nitrogen and low in fibre, and that the character of this diet is responsible for many of the life-threatening and degenerative illnesses that afflict us. I am interested in taking this argument one stage further. If the average diet was miraculously altered in line with the nutritionists' ideal, would people's health problems disappear? In my opinion, they would not. Health problems would undoubtedly be reduced, but they would not disappear. We have to gain a deeper understanding of the food we eat.

Take it as a given that we should strive to avoid processed, refined or non-organic foods. These foods do not aid the digestion. All raw foods contain the enzymes necessary for their digestion. Processing techniques and cooking are estimated to destroy 100 per cent of these enzymes. Even in raw food there are fewer enzymes than there once were, because of the nutrient-depleted soil in which it is grown and the techniques used to keep food looking 'fresh' and supermarket bright. The problem of our internal enzyme production reducing with age, illness, stress, pregnancy, exercise, cold weather and over-consumption of caffeine and alcohol is compounded by these external factors. An enzyme deficient body plus enzyme-deficient food places a burden on the digestive system that it was not designed to shoulder.

We should strive to balance our intake of organic foods, with vegetables and fruit predominating. In addition, we should pay attention to freshness when selecting fruit, vegetables and dried food. If food looks tired and as though it has been sitting on a shelf for a lifetime, it will probably have tiny fungi growing on it. Once ingested these may contribute to an existing overgrowth of bacteria in the gut. The vitamin and mineral benefits found in vegetables and fruit also rapidly diminish once they have been removed from the soil or cut from the plant.

However, as will become clear from the individual programmes, even ostensibly valuable foods in terms of their nutritional content are not good for us in all circumstances.

- Bread, for example – even that made perfectly with organic whole-wheat flour – is one of the most difficult of all foods to digest properly, because it is a starch with a high gluten content and requires acid in quantities most people cannot muster to break it down.
- Pulses invariably do not do as much good as they should because they are so difficult to digest.
- Raw vegetables are wonderful if the digestion is right and they are chewed to perfection. If neither of these requirements is met, eating them can be like putting a match to a can of kerosene – the air from them is enough to 'blow up' the whole digestive system.
- Milk and cheese are rich sources of calcium, but for the constipated person with an acid stomach they are wholly inappropriate because they cannot be absorbed and they will block the arteries. Most people find it easier to break down the protein in the milk of goats and ewes. (See Milk, page 137.)
- Potato contains Vitamin C as well as useful amounts of thiamine and nicotinic acid. It also promotes alkalinity. An all-round ideal food, one might think. However, if it is not chewed very well, in some people the starch in cooked potato can go through the stomach lining and raise the glucose level in the blood too much. This has the effect of making the system acid. People with diabetes mellitus and arthritis should not eat potatoes for this reason.

We need to look very carefully at the sources we use to supply our nutritional requirements and learn to select foods that are right for us – this means, foods that are right for the particular state we are in and foods that lighten the load on the system. (See the lists of acid-forming and alkali-forming foods on page 62.)

Watering the Body

One vital element of diet that is often overlooked is our intake of water. Alcohol, tea, coffee and soft drinks are not substitutes for this essential component. Water is needed for every bodily function. Without it enzymes and nutrients could not be transported around the body. It helps to dilute acids, makes the blood more alkaline, helps the kidneys excrete acids and us to digest nutrients, and provides moisture for the skin.

A sure sign that we are not drinking enough water is the condition of the skin. In a well-watered body this will be soft to the touch. In a dehydrated body it will look dry and wrinkly.

There is a debate about what sort of water is best: tap, mineral or distilled. Distilled water, it is claimed, is the purest type of water available, because it contains none of the poisons, pollutants or inorganic mineral substances found in tap and mineral water. For those with sufficient time and enthusiasm, it is possible to steam-distil your own water at home with the appropriate equipment. However, this is not necessary. It is far better to drink the correct volume of water from a less than pure source than to be dehydrated. We know that chronic dehydration can be a contributory factor in asthma, high blood pressure, heartburn, indigestion, fatigue, backache and pains in the joints, that it exacerbates the effects of constipation, and that it allows toxins to crystallize into gall stones, whereas the jury is still out on the respective merits or dangers of the different types of water.

In order to do its good work water must stay in the body long enough to circulate and wash away waste matter. Traditional drinks such as tea and coffee promote the elimination of urine and thus do not perform this function.

Try to drink between 1.5–2 litres ($2^1/_2$–$3^1/_2$ pints) of water per day, 3 litres (5 pints) if you are constipated. I cannot pretend that drinking this amount of water every day is unalloyed pleasure – a disguise is necessary. My favourite water-based drink is made of lemon:

Take a mug, put a couple of slices of organic lemon and a generous squeeze of the juice in it and then fill with boiling water.

Lemon is wonderfully cleansing and alkalizing. Alternatives are to add a knob or two of fresh ginger or try herb or fruit teas. Eating foods that are high in water, such as fruit and vegetables, will also help your intake of healthy liquids.

Monitoring the amount you drink can be problematic. I find that I have either to get into a routine or post reminders to myself. Each night before I go to bed, I put a pint mug next to the kettle so that in the morning the sight of it prompts me to make that first cleansing drink of the day.

Which Values?

Many people, especially women, tend to look at food in terms of calorific values, because weight is their primary concern. My primary concern is helping people to attain good health through a robust digestive system. It makes no sense, for example, to choose to eat cheese rather than avocado. On the face of it cheese has fewer calories, but avocado is far and away the better food nutritionally. A food that is difficult to digest, such as cheese, will ferment badly and eventually show itself as extra weight. Excess weight denotes toxins the body could not cope with. We have already had the example of the man who ate nothing but lettuce and still gained weight (see page 31). Excess volume and poor digestion were the causes of his misery. Take another example.

A woman with bad migraines came to me. I suggested which foods she should eat and which she should avoid, and gave her some drops. She went on holiday and lost one stone in a week. She came back, quickly resumed her stressful lifestyle, and within days had put on five pounds after eating one cream cracker. She thought such an innocuous food could not harm her because it had no calories. That cream cracker would have made no difference to her weight if she had eaten it when she was calm and relaxed. However, by eating it when she was stressed, she blocked her digestion. This shock brought home to her the necessity of regarding the act of eating as one of the most important rituals in life and according it the respect it deserves.

If we get the acid balance right in the digestion, we will be healthier and slimmer. The calorific value of foods is irrelevant to this process. Slimmers on low-calorie diets have been found to put on weight relative to those on a diet that is high in fruit, vegetables and slow-release carbohydrates. How we break down our food has more to do with our weight than the number of calories we consume. The ability of the body to make the right digestive enzymes is often a factor in weight-related problems, as is low blood sugar syndrome. If the blood sugar is not kept even by means of a diet that is high in fibre, vegetables and other slow-release foods (for example, oats and millet), the glucose response at the top of the 'swing' – when something sweet or a stimulant, such as coffee, has been taken – will result in the excess blood sugar being turned into fat.

Some patients of mine with so-called weight problems have reduced their clothes size significantly without losing a pound. The body will start to change shape if the digestive system is functioning correctly. In order to get this right, we must – in addition to mastering the basics of volume, chewing and relaxing (see page 28) – learn to select our foods on the basis of how easy they are to digest and how beneficial they are in respect of the bacterial flora.

Pathway 3 – EXERCISE

Exercise is just one component among the several factors that keep us healthy. Little or no physical activity does not encourage the body to eliminate impurities, hence the digestion becomes sluggish and the person constipated. Some people get so little exercise that shopping at the supermarket on Saturday morning is the closest they get to working up a sweat. However, before you rush out to exercise madly, and distance yourself from those lazy people whose trolleys are undoubtedly heaving with refined carbohydrates, consider.

Getting Physical

Used unwisely, exercise can be positively harmful. Many people talk of exercising to get in shape. They would be better advised to get in shape first, by clearing up the body on the inside, and then exercising. A person with arthritis does not have to run miles to get their circulation moving. Although it is not a good idea to do a lot of nothing, equally we should not do too much of anything without appropriate preparation. Spring is a wonderfully lucrative time for chiropractors and osteopaths as all those winter house-bound gardeners and sportsmen rush enthusiastically into action, only to be laid low by the first day's digging or game.

A toxic body is a stiff body which stores in its tissues what it cannot cope with, either as cellulite or oily patches. Toxic tissue is like sandpaper – things adhere to it. A toxic person who sits in a draught will get a stiff neck. If you were to run in a toxic body, your limbs would become progressively stiffer and eventually force you to stop. We speak of 'running out of steam' – what happens is that we run out of energy, which has been gobbled up by the toxins. When the body clears up on the inside, we do not get stiff.

I am careful not to rush people who come to me feeling very tired. I tell them not to worry about exercise until they feel like doing some. There is no point in forcing a body that is already abused. Find your body first. Give yourself about a month on whichever programme you decide is appropriate, then see how you feel. If you take up an activity, build up slowly and then try to maintain the same level throughout the year. If you want to do more, increase the level gradually to minimize the risk of strain. But never over-do it – ultra-strenuous exercise depresses the immune system. Gentle exercise, on the other hand, such as brisk walking, boosts it. Meditation, massage and laughter significantly raise levels of secretory IgAs, an immune system protein.

Pathway 4 – MEDICATION

From a holistic standpoint, every disease state produces toxic agents – pus is an example of one such toxin – which the body struggles to eliminate through its own defence mechanisms. These mechanisms include antibodies, toxin defence via the nervous system, and detoxification via the liver and the connective tissue. The last-mentioned, for example – the body's generalized cellular tissue – supports the organs, vessels and more specialized cells by acting as a sort of deposition and drainage system, receiving waste matter from the cells and either depositing them or transporting them away via the lymphatic system. Many types of drugs including chemotherapeutic and immunosuppressive substances, antibiotics and salicylates interfere with this process of biological defence and can make the toxin situation in the body worse. Most anti-inflammatory and pain-killing drugs, for example, irritate the gut and cause problems in long-term users.

Antibiotics and a great number of other types of drugs kill off all fermentation with a view to bringing the body under control – the word 'antibiotic' means 'against life'. When you stop taking these drugs it would be a miracle if more good bacteria than bad re-emerged in the gut. A diet high in refined foods and sugar will ensure that they do not.

Drugs can save lives, and when they do we are thankful for them. Too often, however, they are used where gentler, less drastic alternatives would be more beneficial although perhaps slower in producing a result. Societies would be much healthier overall if they could learn to use appropriately the medical means available, conventional or complementary. No one can predict with certainty what effect antibiotics and other medical drugs will have on subsequent generations.

The taking of amphetamines or water pills – usually by people who are trying to lose weight – tends to lead to the production of toxins. The person invariably loses weight, but as soon as the pills are stopped on come the pounds.

The problem with common simple medications such as antacids and headache pills is that they mask what is really going on in the body. In many cases they are short-term solutions. They remind me of bribes given to disruptive or difficult children by desperate or lazy mothers. An antacid tablet, for example, may dispel the acid but in achieving this much it will upset the usual response of the liver and pancreas. The problem – incorrect fermentation – is thus pushed further along in the system to show itself elsewhere, as wind.

If you are taking prescribed drugs, be aware that your body will need help to absorb the vital trace elements it needs. For anyone undergoing radical treatment, such as chemotherapy, it is important to take as many trace elements as possible without upsetting the stomach. These can be found in easily absorbable foods such as Green Energy, aloe vera or Cal-M. When the course of treament has finished your body will be tired and will need looking after. Careful eating in combination with a couple of months of taking Acidophilus tablets should help to balance the bacterial flora in the gut. Once the bacterial flora are balanced, the body will be able to absorb nutrients in the usual way.

Pathway 5 – STRESS

The usual caricature of a stressed person is one of the headless chicken tendency we met earlier in this chapter – someone who is always on the go, never has enough time, and does not know the meaning of the word 'relax'. Stress can take many forms, and in some of these passivity is a hallmark in which the stress works away so quietly it goes almost unnoticed or by another name. Anxiety and anger have a negative effect on the gut and the microflora within it, raising the level of insulin in the blood and causing even good food to become toxic. In some people the toxins may clog the arteries and cause heart problems. The adverse effects of negative emotions on the body are well understood in Chinese medicine, which identifies emotional stress and pain as interfering with the proper functioning of the body's organs. Excessive anger, for example, harms the liver's ability to store blood and can bring on headaches, premenstrual tension or irregular periods. Many types of behaviour can stress the homeostasis, or natural balance, of the body. We can stress ourselves by eating the wrong types of food (for us). Constipation is a form of stress, as is over-eating or a panic attack.

We need to understand ourselves well enough to know where we put our stress. How does your stress manifest itself – in your stomach, your kidneys or your adrenaline? When you are anxious or upset, do you become constipated, wee uncontrollably, have diarrhoea, or get indigestion? An understanding of how we function and react is vital if we are to learn to limit the damage we do to ourselves. The body is like a naughty boy – we have to find ways of keeping him in order or diverting him from mischief. If we keep letting him run away from us, one day he may just turn our lives upside down.

Caring for Ourselves

Many of us are very bad at looking after ourselves in fundamental ways. We may pay attention to cosmetics, and spend time and effort disguising our obvious physical flaws and showing off our best bits, but generally that is as far as we go. We look after our pets better than ourselves. Most of us are like neglected racehorses – we have the potential in our genes, but the work is not being put in to make us winners. No trainer worth his salt would enter a horse for a race without getting it in tip-top condition first, through diet, exercise and general tender loving care. Afterwards he would be just as diligent, resting him until the time was right to start building him up for the next race. And so it should be with us.

Modern life demands a lot. That is fine so long as we make sure we replenish our stocks of mental, physical and spiritual energy. For various reasons, there is a tendency for people to give more than is good for their health. Some people may not realize the amount which they are taking out of themselves until they are forced to, for example by illness. If we want to be healthy, we have at some point to examine the way we are living and begin to take responsibility in a very basic sense on our own account in order to achieve our goal.

It is surprising how many people unconsciously live to someone else's design. They will put the well-being of everyone else in their lives – parents, spouse or partner, children, friends – before their own. A patient of mine, who suffered with arthritis from a relatively young age, did precisely that. Even in illness he put his nearest and dearest first, to the point where he jeopardized his life. He knew all about hard work, duty, obligations. He knew nothing about fun or pleasing himself.

We owe it to our real selves not to be too nice, too unselfish. If we always behave as others want us to, there is a danger of us ending up fulfilling their dreams and not our own. Once I got my patient to understand this (and it took me getting very angry and shocking him), he looked at his life afresh and began to take a genuine interest in getting better for his own sake. His condition has improved in leaps and bounds, and I am confident that together we will keep it under control in future.

At some point in our lives we have to discover what makes us happy and start saying 'No' to what does not. If we are not happy, we lay ourselves wide open to physical illness. Those who genuinely believe, as did my patient, that they can expect little for themselves should perhaps reflect on the Buddhist idea of care: only by looking after ourselves in all respects are we able to help others.

Living for Ourselves

We have to learn the art of living for our real selves. This does not mean working ten hours a day to increase our social standing or purchasing power. Work is important, but it should not be allowed to dominate. A successful life is made up of many dimensions, of which work is only one. To be healthy in all senses, we need to strike a balance between the mental, the physical and the spiritual, the public and the private. Imagine a lifestyle in which each day you spent four or five hours working, two or three hours meditating and assimilating your experiences, and between two and four hours in joyful pursuits of your own choosing.

That sort of balance might seem like a Utopian dream, but it is one worth aspiring to. Feudalism died out in the Middle Ages and yet in some important respects we are no more liberated now than we were then. It is important to build time into our lives; time to allow us those 'free' spaces to breathe, and not to become complete victims of circumstances. Each day steal those moments for yourself, even if it means disappearing into the loo at work periodically.

At lunchtime, instead of rushing off to shop or queuing for a sandwich, use this time for yourself. Prepare a lunch box before you leave home in the morning (or the night before), go to a quiet place, sit down and savour the time you have away from work (see page 58). At the end of the day, reflect, assimilate your experiences and learn from them. Life is precious; it is a gift; it is short; and it is yours. Ask yourself what you want. Even if the answer you come up with seems like a pipe dream, do not discard it. Treasure it, concentrate your inner energies on finding ways of making it become a reality.

Chapter Three

PATHWAYS TO REGENERATION

Few of my patients believe me when I tell them that clearing their bodies and getting their digestions right will change them in unsuspected ways. A mind living in a clear body is a dimension away from one living in a toxic body. After a couple of weeks people begin to feel differently, and after three months many would not recognize themselves. Living in a clear body is like perpetually feeling as you would after a relaxing holiday – happier, kinder, more thoughtful.

Pathway 1
– THE NATURE OF ILLNESS

Health and happiness go hand in hand. Even small chronic afflictions reduce our capacity for life and undermine our self-confidence. In each of us there is a tendency to live through our problems. We may ignore them in the hope they will go away; dismiss them as trifling; use them as a means of attracting attention; or develop them as a form of punishment. Each of these approaches represents a form of acceptance.

Escape Routes

I had one patient who would arrive at every dinner party with about twenty different sorts of vitamins, pills and potions. She would sit down at the table with the other guests and pull out her battery of medicines. Naturally, everybody else would stop what they were talking about and focus on the woman and her medicines. When I pointed out to her subsequently that there was no need for her to take them all with her, she said, 'Gudrun, I can only do it this way.'

This woman used what appeared to be an obsession with her health as a form of escapism, to put her centre stage and convince herself – if only for a few hours – that life was worth living. Work or dangerous hobbies can fulfil a similar function for other people. One of the most common escape routes is the bread bin or a bumper box of chocolates. When we dive into either of them we are saying we do not want to look at our lives. Dwelling in either for too long eventually exhausts the body's energy and makes clear thinking an impossibility. At some point during the drive through life most of us have found ourselves screaming on the back seat, hating the journey but seemingly incapable of changing the route. Wherever we are in our lives we must try not to undermine our health, and thus our potential for happiness, by being our own worst enemy.

Millstones

Bad situations with our health can arise out of circumstances which we arrange for ourselves. One classic example of this presented itself in a single working mother who came to me with her two-year-old daughter. The child was glowing with health. The mother, who is a hyper-personality type, said she felt like a lead weight and had no energy. The cause of her malaise quickly became apparent.

Since the child's birth she had given it all her attention, taking it everywhere, having it sleep in the same bed, and allowing it to suckle throughout the night. All was fine while the child's means of expression was limited to baby babble, but when this developed into an identifiable vocabulary the mother was horrified to hear the child demanding loudly in public what it had grown used to enjoying in private. Regularly she would flee from a restaurant or shop with the accompanying shout of 'I want mummy's titty' ringing in her embarrassed ears. By the time she came to me, she had reached the stage where she dared not take the child out in public.

As I saw the situation, my task was to release the woman from the prison she had built for herself. I got her to realize that by transferring her energy to the child she had left nothing for herself. If she was to avoid becoming ill, she had to start looking after herself and stop over-mothering.

Low Blood Sugar Blues

A high proportion of my patients – and I dare say people in general – suffer from hypoglycaemia, most of them without realizing. When I tell someone they have low blood sugar, their usual response is a slightly miffed 'But I'm not diabetic!'. Then they proceed to assure me that liking sweets and being starving every afternoon is part of their make-up – they have always been like this. I do not dispute these facts for one minute, but they do not alter the necessity for a reappraisal.

For the effects of hypoglycaemia to be felt, your blood sugar does not have to fall below the clinical defining line. The vast majority of sufferers will fall between the baseline and the normal level, and many of them will be only just below that normal level. People who present to their doctors with hypoglycaemic symptoms (typically, mood swings, lack of thirst, the tendency to over-indulge and be hyper) and yet pass the blood sugar test are often told that they are suffering from stress or hysteria.

If you are hypoglycaemic, even only mildly, this needs to be taken into account when clearing the body. If you are almost certain that you are not, although you admit to liking sweet foods and starches and having a few other classic symptoms of hypoglycaemia, please turn to page 102 anyway. It may be that after reading the text on Low Blood Sugar you will change your mind or recognize the signs in your partner, a friend, one of your children or even a parent. Low blood sugar is one of the great potential health spoilers, and it need not be.

What's in a Name?

Every medical problem you can think of – including allergies – comes about because the body has been put under stress. I make no distinction between allergies and other forms of illness because, in my experience, they spring from the same single source. Allergies normally start off with indigestion or bloating and belching as a result of food sitting in the stomach too long. An allergy – whether it be a rash, a headache, indigestion or osteo-arthritis – is a trigger which could not be pulled if the fermentation in the gut was correctly balanced. Your trigger may not be the same as someone else's – hence your condition will be called by one name and theirs by another – but the underlying cause will be the same.

According to Dr Anders Hoys, whose clinic in Copenhagen developed the ELISA (Enzyme Linked Immuno Sorbant Assay) test for Helicobacter and IgG (Ig means 'immunoglobulin') food intolerance, 'every food is a potential antigen if it is not correctly broken down by the digestive system. If it is sufficiently broken down by the digestive system, then any food, however potentially toxic, will pass into the lymph system without adverse response'. In people with high levels of Ig the 'pond' in the gut is anaerobic, meaning that the conditions are right for the wrong bacteria to flourish. One of the world's leading allergy specialists, Dr James Braly, also supports the connection between 'allergies' and leaky gut. He has cited large molecules of incompletely digested food entering the bloodstream via holes in the wall of the small intestine as the starting point of allergies.

In most cases of so called food intolerance the person with the allergy sets about trying to identify the substance or food that is causing the problem with the aim of excluding it from their diet. Some people get to the stage with this method where there is virtually nothing left for them to eat because so much has to be excluded. Merely to avoid the food or foods is not the answer. Unless the underlying fermentation problem is addressed, another trigger will simply replace the one or ones removed, and the problem will continue. The questions to ask are: How am I digesting this food? and Why is this food giving me difficulty?. Interestingly, the difficult-to-digest foods or substances – such as gluten, cow's milk, monosodium glutamate, food colourings – are the ones that crop up time and again as the culprits in allergy tests. These also just happen to be the most acid-forming foods.

If the fermentation is not right, if there is not enough hydrochloric acid in the stomach, if food is not chewed properly, then, in the case of a person who eats a great deal of bread which needs that particular acid to break it down, an allergic reaction, such as cystitis, will develop. If your system is acidic and you eat foods with a high sugar content, you will develop skin problems or experience mood swings. If the fermentation is right and the alkaline/acid balance is correct along the length of the digestive tract, the likelihood of your becoming ill (allergic) is greatly reduced.

In my files I have numerous examples of people with so called allergies who have benefited from putting their digestion right. Here are two of them.

One patient could not sit in his garden because of the severity of his hay fever. We worked together on his digestion for over a year during which time he started to change shape and feel much better in himself. His hay fever has now diminished as a problem to the point where he can comfortably sit in his garden.

Another patient used to get severe skin irritations if she ate anything other than pears or lamb. As a result of changing the bacterial flora in her system and making her digestion function as it should, she began to reintroduce foods successfully and can now even eat bread without provoking a reaction. She used to be what I would call a totally allergic person, but she can now cope because her digestion is better.

In neither case did I treat the symptoms. I dealt with what I consider to be the underlying problem in most disease states – incorrect fermentation in the gut.

Changing the Blueprint

Instead of accepting or embracing our ailments, we should ask why we have them, and search for possible reasons. Undoubtedly we inherit a predisposition or tendency towards certain illnesses. When most people say matter-of-factly, 'Oh, we always suffer from asthma'; or 'We always suffer from arthritis'; or 'The men always lose their hair', the inference is that the condition is unavoidable. We are, to a greater or lesser extent, either handicapped by our genetic inheritance or benefited by it. The body has its own memory, and our cells carry a record of our ancestors and what afflicted them.

Asthma, for example, can be seen as a specific response to toxic overload programmed into the blueprint of a child in whom the barrier protecting against such an overflow has been breached. An infant born of a mother who has taken a great many courses of antibiotics will inherit her weakened immune system. Any physical deficiency in a child-bearing mother will find its way into her offspring, initially via the umbilical cord and later through the milk. It takes several generations to clean a line of physical weakness: if TB is in a family, weakness in the lungs will be seen in descendants for several generations; the babies of thalidomide sufferers are now having children with abnormalities.

However, just as the person with a strong constitution can undermine it with constant abuse, so the person who has drawn a meaner health straw can nurture theirs and, with perserverance, overcome shortcomings. It is possible to alter even an unfavourable genetic pattern for the better or ameliorate the worst aspects of that pattern. Although the brain in the large intestine (see page 14) carries the memory of familial weakness, we can prevent an inherited tendency from showing itself, by maintaining our buffer and preventing toxins leaking through the gut into an organ.

The first step is to discover the nature of our genetic weakness. Look back in your family and decide whether there is a history of, for example, early heart disease, early breast cancer, diabetes or asthma. Who do you take after? If you do not know, ask your parents or other relatives.

Do your illnesses tend to take a particular form? Are you aware of a weakness in yourself, such as a particular recurring infection?

In some cases our inheritance does us no favours. I was born into a diabetic family, and thus from infancy had a liking for sweets, puddings and starchy foods. In my case this weakness was reinforced by my mother. Every day during my childhood she ensured I had a three-course lunch and a three-course dinner. She would cook the main course virtually to a cinder, and yet produce wonderful desserts. Now I can understand her order of priorities, and her requirement of getting an insulin-lift from the dessert. I learned very early to cook for myself, because, the wondrous puddings apart, I could not stand her cooking. That decision was my saving.

Your findings may be reassuring: long-lived grandparents on both sides of the family, hale and hearty parents and healthy siblings. But still you feel tired, out of sorts much of the time. Why?

The Degeneration Process

Most of us are at a midway point between illness and health. We do not feel quite right and wished we felt better and yet we have no identifiable disease. The body is a great adapter and uncomplainingly will do its best to cope with our thoughtlessness or ignorance. If someone who has smoked for many years suddenly breaks the habit, they will probably get all sorts of illnesses. These are a sign of the body getting back the energy that the nicotine has been depriving it of and throwing out years of accumulating toxins. Many people who boast of never getting a cold are in a state where the body is so tired it cannot react. I look at health as a pattern of cross-roads. At certain cross-roads we may notice one type of discomfort or disease. If we go on and do not put this right, it will crop up again at a later cross-road, probably appearing as something else but almost certainly deriving from that earlier, untreated problem.

The gradual breakdown of the body's health is called 'dysbiosis', meaning a disturbance of the symbiotic balance which nature intended should exist between the various organs and systems of the body; literally, dys means 'faulty', and bios 'life' or 'growth'.

There are several stages, or crossroads, on the journey to serious illness:

- The body starts to malfunction, with the organs showing signs of hyper- or hypo- activity: fatigue, emotional swings, digestive problems.

- Toxins start to build up; the body responds by trying to expel them, through colds, influenza.
- A focus of inflammation is established – for example, in the form of sinusitis, cystitis or colitis.
- Microbial toxins from this focus are released, causing the body to respond inappropriately – symptoms such as hayfever, asthma and eczema appear.
- Toxins and waste products gather, resulting in rheumatism, arthritis and circulatory problems.
- Toxicity increases to a level at which the cells cannot keep healthy and they turn cancerous.

Throughout our lives the body attempts to keep healthy and in balance, often despite our worst unconscious efforts to make it otherwise. When the stresses we impose on it become too severe or prolonged it adapts by becoming ill. Headaches or sinus problems are the body's way of telling us that it is in trouble, and the longer we go on taking short-term relief in pills and medicines the more toxins we are storing up for ourselves and the more serious the disorder will become. If it is a constant feature, even a fact of life as innocuous as wind constitutes a step along the path to degeneration. It is a sign that the digestive system is over-flowing and not working as it should. In many cases only a few simple steps need be taken in order for regeneration to occur.

Pathway 2 – RESTORING THE BALANCE

One of the worst aspects of toxicity is the way it reduces us and makes us less than we were. Doing becomes harder until nothing can be begun without stimuli of some kind, perhaps the fear of the boss's anger or the nagging of a friend to generate sufficient adrenaline or enthusiasm. Most of us need the stimulus of other people to lift us out of our inertia. We all know people who will resist the idea of going out by putting up obstacles but once prised away from home they will be great company, the life and soul of any gathering. These activated couch potatoes are relying on the energy of others to lift them out of their usual semi-supine state. For many people the worst aspect of being alone is the instant 'droop' they experience.

Clearing the system allows us to refill our inner reservoir of energy. The really in-tune person is naturally sociable and yet has the self-confidence and peace of mind to be alone happily. As we become less toxic, energy is used as a harmonizing agent and not as a drug to boost us in social situations.

Assessing the System

The body reacts to faulty digestion in different ways, depending on the genetic blueprint of the individual and the location of their specific health weak spot.

When someone first comes to me I can usually tell what shape they are in from their appearance – their eyes, the way they hold themselves, limb shape and colouring tell me more than the often guarded words of the individual concerned. I will then assess them further by testing the energy levels on the various meridian points in their body with a machine called a biotron. The deficiency of energy at any one of these points will tell me where the problem lies.

Obviously, you cannot be expected to do this for yourself. What you are capable of doing, however, is deciding how you feel, listening to what your body is telling you, and assessing yourself honestly.

Answer the following questions –

Are you constipated?

In my experience, few people are initially willing to admit to constipation as a problem. For some reason I have yet to fathom, most people need to feel as normal as possible where bowel movements are concerned. You should go to the lavatory twice a day. See the programme for constipation on page 75, then follow the Basic Programme on page 55.

Do you require certain conditions to enable you to go to the lavatory? What happens when you travel?

'I am not constipated. After my second cup of coffee/third cigarette I always go.' If you need one or two cups of coffee or one, two or three cigarettes to get your system moving each morning, you are constipated. If an upset to your routine blocks your bowel movement, you are constipated. See the programme for constipation on page 75, then follow the Basic Programme on page 55.

Do you get wind or feel bloated?

If your answer is 'No more than the next person', think again. Even discreet wind at either end or bloating signifies a lack of digestive enzymes, especially hydrochloric acid, and a build-up of undigested matter in the system. When these meet the remnants of your previous meal in the system, the results will be explosive. Eating too much, gulping your food and not chewing it thoroughly, perhaps because you are stressed, will block the digestion and cause bloating. A high intake of starch over several days will blow you out; for example, a daily pattern of breakfasting on a pile of toast, waffles or cereals high in sugar and then lunching on a sandwich or two. Switch to non-wheat or low-sugar cereal for breakfast, or, better still, fruit. Alternatively, you could combine the two, accompanying the cereal with some cooked apple, which reduces the tendency to bloat. For lunch, try to break the sandwich mould and have a salad, avocado or cooked vegetables instead. In general, follow the Basic Programme.

Do you get tired in the afternoon?
If you do, you are not digesting your food perfectly and your system is becoming toxic. Short chain carbohydrates (for example, highly refined, sugary foods such as biscuits) are easily absorbed through the stomach lining. The lymphatic in the small intestine needs to be fed too, however. If proteins are fermenting badly and are not broken down properly, they cannot be absorbed in sufficient amounts to nourish the system. Usually the effects of this sort of maldigestion do not become apparent until we reach middle age. Your energy level will not fluctuate as much when your digestion improves and you start to absorb through the small intestine as well as the stomach.

Are you often depressed (seemingly for no good reason), ravenously hungry and tend to over-indulge a weakness for starchy foods, such as biscuits and chocolates?
Turn to page 102.

Do you tend towards diarrhoea?
Diarrhoea is the body's mechanism for getting rid of substances that are irritating the gut wall. Follow the Basic Programme on page 55, but also see page 96.

Does hunger return shortly after you have eaten?
If it does, you are eating too quickly and not chewing your food properly. Eating small meals at regular intervals and taking digestive enzymes should help. Follow the Basic Programme.

Is your stomach acid?
If you have an acid stomach, undigested food is lying too long, it is fermenting badly and the gut lining is irritated. Often the cause is regularly eating too much very quickly. In some sufferers initial low gastric acidity is followed by the over-production of acid. This digestive

system is caught in a vicious spiral – no sooner does it begin to make a small inroad into one load of undigested matter than another helping arrives on top to overwhelm it. A complete change in eating habits and diet is required to clear this build up.

An acid stomach is common among vegetarians because of their high consumption of starch, which, as we have seen, is very difficult to digest. If food is chewed well, and the worst of the acid-forming foods (see page 62) are eliminated from the diet there will be nothing in the system to irritate the stomach and the lining will heal. Follow the Basic Programme on page 55.

Do you never feel thirsty?
One of the reasons why many people drink so little water is because they do not feel thirsty. This phenomenon is one of the classic signs of low blood sugar (see page 102).

Cleaning Up the System

Whatever you discover about your family's health history, or know about your own, the first line of defence for your body is to get the digestion working well. If toxins are not put into the system or manufactured within it, the body will not come under pressure.

The first step in any of my treatments is to exclude from the diet any foods or beverages that are very difficult to digest. Principally these are acid-forming foods. The more severe the condition the longer the list of exclusions, as will be gathered from the individual treatment programmes. However, I recommend for exclusion only what is strictly necessary. I try not to put my patients off before they have begun – the sheer tedium associated with many so-called 'special diets' virtually dooms them to failure. In most cases the exclusions are not permanent. Once the gut flora are flourishing again, foods can in most cases be reintroduced.

If you have a perfect digestive system you can eat whatever you like, in whatever combination and not suffer any ill effects. If, however, you have a weak digestive system, you must look very carefully at what you eat and how you combine foods. Starches, and particularly those containing gluten, are without doubt the most difficult foods for us to digest properly. If we ate small helpings of them and chewed them to perfection, they would be pre-digested in the mouth before they began the long descent through the rest of the digestive system, and far fewer people would have problems with their digestion. Because we cannot be relied upon to be this sensible, we have to find other ways of helping ourselves.

One of the simplest and most effective ways of achieving this is to adopt the method known as food combining; also called the Hay System, after the first man to advocate it, the American medic Dr William Hay. As we have already seen, starches and proteins are incompatible in that they are processed by the body in different ways. By not mixing them at the same meal, the load on the system is automatically lightened.

FOOD COMBINING

The essence of food combining is not to mix protein and starch; for example, meat and potatoes or fish and rice should not be taken at the same meal. You should always aim to eat 4–5 times as much vegetables at either a protein or starch meal. In the following table the foods in columns 1 and 2 or 2 and 3 can be combined. The foods in columns 1 and 3 can not be combined.

COLUMN 1	COLUMN 2	COLUMN 3
FOR PROTEIN MEALS	**NEUTRAL FOODS**	**FOR STARCH MEALS**
Proteins	**Nuts**	**Cereals**
Meat of all kinds: beef, lamb, pork, venison	All except peanuts	Wholegrain: wheat, barley, maize (corn), oats, millet, rice (brown, unpolished), rye.
Poultry: chicken, duck, goose, hare	**Fats**	Bread: 100% wholemeal
Fish of all kinds including shellfish	Butter, cream, egg yolks, olive oil (virgin)	Flour: 100% or 85%
Eggs	Sunflower seed oil (cold pressed)	Oatmeal: medium
Cheese		**Vegetables**
Milk: combines best with fruit and should not be served with a meat meal		Potatoes
Yoghurt		Jerusalem artichokes

COLUMN 1

FOR PROTEIN MEALS

Fruits

Apples, apricots (fresh & dried), blackberries, cherries, currants, gooseberries (if ripe), grapefruit, grapes, kiwis, lemons, limes, loganberries, mangoes, melons (best eaten alone as a fruit meal), nectarines, oranges, papayas, pears, pineapples, prunes (occasionally), raspberries, satsumas, strawberries, tangerines

Salad dressings

French dressing made with oil and lemon juice or apple cider vinegar

Cream dressing

Mayonnaise (homemade)

Sugar substitute

Diluted frozen orange juice

For vegetarians

(but not recommended)

Legumes

Lentils

Soya beans

Chick peas

Butter (lima) beans

Pinto beans

Alcohol

Dry red & white wines

Dry cider

COLUMN 2

NEUTRAL FOODS

Vegetables

Asparagus, aubergines (eggplant), beans (all fresh green beans), beetroot, broccoli, brussels sprouts, cabbage, carrots, cauliflower, celery, courgettes, leeks, kohlrabi, marrow, mushrooms, onions, parsnips, peas, spinach, swedes, turnips

Salad stuffs

Avocados, chicory (endive), corn salad, cucumber, fennel, garlic, lettuce, mustard and cress, peppers, (red and green), radishes, spring onions, sprouted legumes, sprouted seeds, tomatoes (uncooked), watercress

Herbs & Flavourings

Chives, mint, parsley, sage, tarragon, grated lemon rind, grated orange rind

Seeds

Sunflower, sesame, pumpkin

Bran

Oat bran

Wheatgerm

Sugar substitute

Honey

Maple Syrup

Alcohol

Whiskey

Gin

COLUMN 3

FOR STARCH MEALS

Sweet fruits

Bananas (ripe), dates, figs (fresh and dried)

Grapes (extra sweet)

Papaya if very ripe

Pears if very sweet and ripe

Milk & yoghurt

Only in moderation

Salad dressings

Olive oil or cold pressed seed oils.

Fresh tomato juice with oil and seasoning

Sugars

Barbados sugar and honey – in strict moderation

Alcohol

Ale

Beer

Basic Programme

The following programme forms the basis of all my treatments, and it will become the basis of your ongoing self-help campaign to better health. It benefits most people because it shows how to reduce the pressure on any weaknesses, whether these are known to the individual or not.

Look, honestly, at how much you are eating. If at each sitting the amount exceeds what can be contained in your two cupped hands (see page 31), you are eating too much and overloading your system. Try to cut back, gradually if need be. You will find that even a relatively small amount of food becomes a great deal more when it is chewed properly.

Assess the composition of each meal. One-third of the volume should be composed of either starch or protein – do not mix these two at the same meal. The remainder should be raw or gently cooked (steamed or stir-fried) vegetables, depending on how far down the fermentation road you have progressed. For example, if raw vegetables give you wind, you are not digesting them well, so avoid them in favour of slightly cooked vegetables.

Chew each mouthful 50 times. You can change how food behaves – even the wrong food – by the way you eat it. If food is chewed to perfection, you transform it and make it easier to digest. Lumps that are not pre-digested with the saliva will ferment more, stirring up the toxins already in the colon and turning alkali-forming foods into acid-forming ones.

Eat slowly. When you are eating on your own, you will have to concentrate twice as hard, because the tendency to want to get the meal over with as quickly as possible is far greater than when you are sharing a meal with others.

Eat three times a day, unless you have a very poor digestive system which would benefit from five small meals per day. Do not miss meals, thereby stressing your body by forcing it to run on adrenaline.

Daily Regime

On waking each morning drink a glass of water to flush your system.

Breakfast – fruit (e.g. apple, papaya, pear, grapefruit) with some fibre (e.g. oat bran, oat bran flakes or oat flakes), topped with goat or sheep's yoghurt. If you are afflicted with wind, it is better to cook the bran (as porridge) with a whole apple grated into it.

Go to the lavatory. If you have difficulty, use one of the old-fashioned flushers (see page 58). If you are badly constipated (i.e. you go to the toilet once every few days), follow the programme for constipation on page 75.

Lunch – starch (e.g. millet, brown rice, or pasta made from buckwheat or millet, and quinoa) or protein (preferably chicken or fish) with sautéed/steamed/stir-fried vegetables or salad.

Dinner – protein or starch with sautéed/steamed/stir-fried vegetables or salad stuffs.

Mid-afternoon – If you eat late at night, have a cup of light soup or vegetable stock mid afternoon so that your energy levels are not at rock bottom when you come to eat your meal.

Supper – If you eat early in the evening (before 6.30 pm), have a cup of light soup, vegetable stock or stewed prunes shortly before you go to bed to keep your blood sugar levels even until breakfast time.

Additional Musts

Take a small dose of Green Energy foods (see page 135) or Missing Link (see page 138) each day to ensure that you are receiving sufficient trace elements and minerals.

Take a mild model Acidophilus tablet (see Probiotics, page 139) every day. This will keep the digestion under control and ensures that toxicity does not build up too much at the lower end of the system. Acidophilus helps the fermentation, makes the stools softer and strengthens the lymphatic membrane around the intestines.

Drink between 1.5–2 litres ($2^1/_2$–$3^1/_2$ pints) of water per day, unless you are constipated, in which case the volume should be increased to 3 litres (5 pints) per day.

Ensure that your diet is high in unsaturated oils – Everybody needs these (see Essential Fatty Acids, page 131).

Exercise each day if you feel up to it. Do a form enjoyable to you which quickens the heartbeat.

Try To's

Drinks – Try to limit your consumption of tea and coffee. If you simply cannot do without either, buy only high quality varieties and serve it in small cups. Japanese or Chinese green tea (see page 135) is a healthier alternative to traditional Indian tea – as are herb or fruit teas – which your digestive system will appreciate much more. On the alcohol front, it is perfectly all right to have a glass or two of wine with a meal. If you prefer whisky or brandy, by all means have a tot. The point is to be moderate. As with food, if you savour what you do have, you will enjoy it more and it will increase in volume with your appreciation.

Meat – Limit your consumption of red meat, such as beef and pork. If you have a passion for grilled or fried meats, have small amounts and eat them Mediterranean-style, by adding olive oil and lemon, or with fresh herbs, such as tarragon, parsley or dill which will aid their digestion. Organic poultry and game birds are leaner and easier on the digestion than red meat.

Fish – With chicken, this is the best form of protein for the digestion. Shellfish are another matter and suitable only for robust digestions, and even then it is wise to eat them in moderation. If you love shellfish, eat them with papaya and a few twists of lime to help you digest them.

Do not forget the Mediterranean principle – This means eating your food in a relaxed, convivial atmosphere, and allowing yourself time to savour it. We are social animals and sharing a meal with others is a happier experience than sitting down by ourselves. Discussing the day's events good-humouredly, or putting the world to rights over a meal, is a civilizing part of life, and one that benefits all age groups. The circumstances in which we eat have a profound effect on the digestive system, and perching in front of the television set or hunching over a book or newspaper while we eat is an unkindness it can do without.

It is undoubtedly more difficult to make each meal special if you usually eat alone, but try. In addition to making sure that what we eat is tasty and nourishing, we can in small ways enhance the pleasure of eating and in so doing generate positive feelings about ourselves. You could marry the food to an aesthetic pleasure, such as using plates, bowls or cutlery that please you, or putting flowers on the table, or listening to a relaxing piece of music while you eat. By inventing our own rituals, we can elevate to its rightful level what has become for so many people a chore.

Old-fashioned Flushers

You should be able to go to the toilet every morning after drinking a mug or glass of something warm (at least room temperature) or directly after breakfast. As well as encouraging a bowel movement, a warm drink in the morning will make the system more alkaline, thus reducing acidity and making arthritis or other joint problems less likely. Here are a few suggestions:

- A glass of warm water.
- A tablespoon of cider vinegar (use the dried form if your system is delicate) in a glass of warm water. This also lifts the blood sugar, which is low at this time of the day. If you cannot bear the taste, add a bit of honey.
- A tablespoon of lemon in a glass of warm water.
- Much more pleasant tasting than any of these is my favourite – fresh root ginger and lemon in hot water.

The Pit Stop Challenge

Initially most people who read this book will probably think that the diet is the most difficult part of the treatments to implement. How, you are probably wondering, am I supposed to follow it when I am at work? I will not repeat what I have said elsewhere about the importance of changing how we view work, time, food and ourselves (see page 42). However, unless we are prepared to look at these afresh with a view to overhauling our habits, no progress can be made. Ask yourself, in all honesty, if what you are being asked to give up is worth defending. Then look at how simple and relatively easy it is to change your eating habits for the better, even while you are at work.

When I used to go out to work, lunch usually consisted of a sandwich or two and perhaps, on a virtuous day, a piece of fruit. More often than not the fruit was sidelined in favour of a packet of comfort, like chocolate, cake or biscuits. If this roughly describes your routine, ask yourself how much you enjoy this type of meal. In all probability, the sensation of temporarily satisfying your hunger pangs will pass for enjoyment. Lunch at work is more a question of a quick pit stop to refuel before we race back to the track for the prescribed number of afternoon laps. Our food scarcely grazes our teeth as it plummets into the digestive tract, and unless adrenaline is keeping our energy high, by mid-afternoon we are dreaming about a little something to keep us revving until we get home. You can do far better than this. All it takes is a bit of forward planning and a willingness to try something different.

Here are a few ideas to get your imagination working and hopefully excite you into a new way of eating at work and perhaps also at home.

- Buy yourself a plastic dish with a clip lid and a wide necked thermos flask. Thus equipped you will be able to take salads to work in the kinder months and thick soups and stews when the weather is chillier or the fancy takes you. If you have low blood sugar the thermos could be used for vegetable stock so that you can keep up your levels of glucose mid-morning and mid-afternoon.
- Sit down and think about the foods you like to eat, bearing in mind that starches and proteins must not be combined – check with the listings on pages 53–54 to remind yourself which foods belong in which category. You will soon remember which foods should not be combined, so do not let the thought of having to double-check put you off.
- Just a word here about starch, which can be a misleading term and one that immediately conjures up visions of bread, rice and potatoes. Starch comes from other sources, too, such as cooked vegetables, although not in such high concentrations. You might find it easier to take a protein lunch to work than a starch one. Here are some protein options: a piece of cold roast chicken, sardines, tuna, mackerel, salmon, goat or ewe's feta cheese, buffalo mozzarella, hard-boiled egg and cold hard roe. I am not in favour of processed food generally, but tinned fish that have not been adulterated with colouring or other chemical agents are perfectly acceptable as well as being quick and easy.
- There are many tasty and nourishing vegetable and salad options to accompany your meat, fish or rice. Gone are the days when lettuce was the only type of salad leaf available. Most supermarkets now stock a wide range of prepared leaves – for example, radicchio, endive, lamb's lettuce, rocket, baby spinach, lollo rosso, tango lettuce, watercress, alfalfa, cress, chervil. Try one or more of these dressed with garlic, extra virgin olive oil, a dash of cider vinegar or lemon and herbs. To them you could also add all kinds of other salad stuffs, such as radishes, celery, chicory, courgettes, avocado and mushrooms. Experiment. Also, try growing sprouting beans,

such as aduki, mung, chickpeas and lentils, or alfalfa at home – it is very simple and will take only a little of your time. All you need is a seed tray, a cover (a piece of cloth will do), somewhere warm and dark to leave it (extremes of temperature or sunlight will leave sprouting beans tasting bitter), and to remember to rinse the sprouts in water once a day. Most sprouting beans (except alfalfa) are wind-forming in most people and should be cooked before they are eaten.

- Get into the habit of cooking more vegetables than you need for dinner and taking them to work the following day, perhaps mixed with rice (red or brown wild rice has a fantastic flavour); similarly, quinoa or millet can form the basis of nourishing salads of this sort. You could also heat the vegetables in the morning and put them in a wide-necked thermos flask. Alternatively, you could fill the thermos with chicken or vegetable stock and take the vegetables cold, dressed with olive oil and lemon. At lunchtime, drink the stock before you eat the vegetables to warm your system and aid digestion.

- In the winter months, try grated raw vegetables, such as turnip, carrot, beetroot (this is also tasty cooked and served cold, dressed with oil and cider vinegar), celeriac (delicious served the French way, raw with a mustard vinaigrette), apple and cauliflower, shredded cabbage (red and white). But do be sure to chew them very well. Remember also to add herbs – these always help the digestion and, of course, will add to the taste of the dish.

- If you feel peckish mid-morning or mid-afternoon, eat fruit. Take different fruits from the ones you have at breakfast – for example, cherries, grapes, figs, dates, mangoes or passion fruit. Alternatively, you could take a pot of home-made fruit salad, yoghurt with honey or cooked apple with honey.

After trying just a few of these options, I shall be very surprised if you do not become hooked. You will probably find, too, that your workmates cast an envious glance or two in your direction. While they are rushing off to queue at the local sandwich bar or office vending machine, you can calmly find some quiet corner where you can tuck into your box of wholesome, tasty food, saving yourself time, money and stress.

Foods and their Traces: Alkali- and Acid-forming Foods

One of the great confusions with food concerns the terms alkaline and acid. Alkaline foods will not make the system alkaline, nor will acid foods make it acid. The reverse is the case.

Foods such as lentils, prunes, brown rice and peas might seem beyond reproach, but each of them leaves an acid ash in the system. It is advisable to eat in moderation those foods liable to leave an acid deposit and eat more of their alkaline counterparts. Many foods we tend to think of as acid – the lemon is probably the classic example – in fact have an alkalizing effect and are beneficial to the good microflora in the digestive system.

There are varying degrees of acidity and alkalinity, of course. For example, figs are the most alkali-forming food, wheat the most acid-forming food; at the other end of the spectrum, apple is among the least alkali-forming of the acid foods and hazel the least acid-forming of the alkaline foods.

Thorough chewing makes food alkaline through the action of the saliva, and if the volume of food at each sitting is small the pepsin and hydrochloric acid will continue this process. So remember: if you chew well and thus digest properly, and you do not overload or stress your system, acid-forming foods will be transformed and do you little harm.

Crisis Management

When toxins start breaking down in the body in response to your change in eating habits, there is danger of the system becoming overloaded with them if sensible precautions are not taken. Such an overload can cause all manner of unpleasant symptoms, from headache to skin eruptions. According to the philosophy that accompanies some therapies, the remedy is not working if the body does not show some sign of this sort. I think it is better to avoid such 'dramas' by taking matters more slowly. If the body is already under stress from the condition itself, it is counter-productive to add to the trauma. Making changes will undoubtedly stir up your system, but in a controlled way. We want to eliminate the 'nasties', not have them running riot inside your body. Whichever programme you follow, be sensible and take it slowly.

In practice this advice sometimes falls on deaf ears. Some of my patients take too much of what I give them in the mistaken belief that

Alkali-Forming Foods

Almonds

Fruit:
- Apples
- Apricots
- Avocados
- Bananas
- Blackberrries
- Cherries, sour
- Dates, dried
- Figs, dried
- Grapefruit
- Grapes
- Lemons
- Limes
- Olives
- Oranges
- Peaches
- Pears
- Pineapple
- Raisins
- Raspberries
- Rhubarb
- Rosehips
- Strawberries
- Tangerines

Herbs

Milk, goat

Millet

Molasses

Pulses:
- Beans, dried
- Lentils, dried
- Lima beans, dried

Salad Stuffs:
- Celery
- Cucumbers
- Dandelion greens
- Lettuce
- Radishes
- Tomatoes
- Watercress

Sauerkraut

Seaweeds

Tofu

Vegetables:
- Beans, green
- Beet greens
- Beets
- Broccoli
- Cabbage
- Carrots
- Cauliflower
- Chard leaves
- Garlic
- Ginger
- Leeks
- Lima beans, green
- Mushrooms (including Shitake)
- Onions
- Parsnips
- Peas, green
- Potatoes, sweet
- Potatoes, white
- Spinach, raw
- Squash

Acid-Forming Foods

Bread:
- White
- Wholewheat

Carob

Cereals:
- Barley
- Bran (wheat and oat)
- Oatmeal
- Rice (white, brown, wild)
- Rye
- Wheatgerm

Chocolate

Coffee

Crackers (soda)

Dairy:
- Cheese
- Cream
- Milk
- Yoghurt

Eggs

Fat:
- Butter
- Margarine

Flour (white and wholewheat)

Fruit:
- Plums
- Pomegranates
- Prunes

Liquor

Meat:
- Bacon
- Beef
- Lamb
- Pork
- Veal

Mayonnaise

Nuts:
- Hazel
- Brazil
- Walnut
- etc.

Pasta:
- Macaroni
- Spaghetti
- etc.

Peanuts
- Peanut butter

Poultry:
- Chicken
- Turkey
- etc.

Seafood:
- Fish
- Shellfish

Sunflower seeds

Tea

Vegetables:
- Asparagus
- Beans, brown
- Corn
- Horseradish
- Peas, dried

it will make them better more quickly. I can understand the temptation. Many years ago, when I was interested in the superficial aspects of health, I read a book called *How to Keep Younger Forever*. This advised readers on how to get sufficient amounts of a DNA component that was said to contain youth-maintaining properties. The main sources of this substance, it told me, were beetroot, fish (specifically sardines) and alfalfa seeds. I plunged headlong into a dietary regime consisting of liberal quantities of sardines and alfalfa seeds, and one pint of freshly pressed beetroot juice. I was sick for three days. Nowhere had the author of that book told me to drink one pint of beetroot juice. I had arbitrarily decided on that amount because I had been told it was a good thing to drink.

This experience has taught me to be very careful when advising other people about their treatments and to point out the dangers of being too 'busy'. The body does not start to clear up until the third day of any treatment at which point it starts to eat up supplies in the body, i.e. the toxins. You can dilute these toxins and the side-effects they can produce by ensuring that you drink a lot of water (2–3 litres/ $3^1/2$–5 pints per day).

Pathway 3 – CHANGE

The digestion can be very difficult to change. It is like a stubborn old horse or dog (or person for that matter), set in its ways and defying you to teach it something different. You will have to trick it until it starts feeling better, usually after two or three months, when it will positively enjoy being treated in the new-fangled way. Most people who persevere with the Basic Programme reach the stage where the body will object if they treat it otherwise or revert to their old habits. Your confidence in your body and your ability to turn round any health problem will increase in line with your strength and vitality.

When the body is introduced to change it does not get better and better, but swings like a pendulum. These swings gradually become less dramatic until the body achieves equilibrium. For example, you may experience two good days followed by a bad day, then three good days followed by a bad one, and so on until all your days are good.

Some patients at first resist the idea of being put on a diet, because they equate diet with weight loss. The sole point of the diet, however, is to reduce toxicity. Any weight loss or change of shape that occurs is incidental. One very over-weight asthma sufferer came to me asking for help. When I told her that I wanted to change her diet, she resisted strenuously, saying 'I don't want to lose weight. I'm beautiful as I am'. She took a great deal of convincing that a change of body shape would not mean that she need think less of herself. When people are asked to do or think differently, often they have to confront deep-seated insecurities or assumptions about themselves and their lives. This is not easy, and acceptance may take some time.

Some people never manage to clear this hurdle. I have one patient who will not give up sugar, although she is overweight and arthritic. This woman has a responsible job and is well educated and yet she refuses to understand that the sugar makes her acidic and that until she cuts it out of her diet she will not get better. The need to have her daily fix is greater than her desire to be well.

The necessity to re-assess does not stop when people are feeling better in themselves and good about the treatment. A patient who had come to me suffering from exhaustion commented one day: 'I'm so pleased. I have so much energy, I can now play tennis in the middle of the night'. The fact that he had now swung into hyperactivity certainly did not please me. I had to explain that the point of his treatment was not to enable him to 'race' his body – continuing along that path would soon bring him back to square one. In order to remain well he would have to look at life differently and see that his new-found energy would have to be used responsibly if it was to benefit him in the long term. Reading, cooking a meal, meditating or strolling in the country or by the sea take energy, as do talking, thinking or entertaining. Strenuous pursuits such as mountaineering, cross-country skiing, or beating an opponent at some game or other are not the only uses worthy of it. The well person very often wears their healthiness lightly and does not need to show it off.

Entering the Straight and Narrow

Change is never easy, and the hardest part of what I do involves getting a person on the 'right' path and then encouraging them to stick to it. Many people almost defy me to help them, and put up obstacles. This may sound illogical, because they are paying for my expertise and yet at the same time seemingly trying to frustrate my best efforts. Sometimes I cannot help feeling that this process is as much a test of my professionalism as of their resolve. Persuasion is thus a key tool of my trade.

Putting into action a strategy for taking care of ourselves can be almost as difficult as finding one in the first place. Unless you are very determined and strong-willed, you will inevitably on occasions find yourself straying from what is best for your body. Expect this to happen, and be relaxed about it when it does. All of us are ridiculous when we try to bend the rules to make them a little more palatable. Learn to laugh at yourself. When we slip there is a tendency to take out our frustration on ourselves. 'It's not working', we say in exasperation, and then throw the regime out of the window. This usually happens when we have tried to be too 'good' and the strain has become intolerable. We are expecting too much of ourselves. None of my patients is a saint or likes the idea of lying on a bed of nails, and I am constantly being challenged to find ways of change that are acceptable to them.

Discover what you are prepared to do. There are limits, obviously. Change does not occur by itself. The individual has to be involved in the process and help it. Try not to think of caring for your body as something to be endured. Look at it positively as something you want to do. In the beginning it is likely you will only half-believe this, but try to convince yourself anyway. Put yourself in charge of what you are doing. Your body is yours, not someone else's.

Trick Not Treat

Trying to do anything new and different teaches us a great deal about ourselves. A bit of humility, a sense of humour, and a little inventiveness will help you cope magnificently. Trick yourself, if need be. If, for example, you are the sort of person who will get through countless glasses of wine at a dinner party without even noticing, place a glass of water nearest your drinking hand and position the glass of wine away from it. If you have a very sweet tooth which you have great difficulty not indulging, be honest with yourself and look at ways of keeping temptation out of your way. A sensible preventative would be not to keep stores of sweets or chocolates in the house. If you need a snack mid-afternoon otherwise you become a gibbering, snappy wreck, accept this as a routine but pre-empt the possibility of your falling on sweets or biscuits out of desperation. Plan ahead by having something tasty but non-carbohydrate at home or in the office to see you through.

Lying to ourselves or pretending to take one course of action while in fact following another can be self-damaging. One very large former patient of mine could not understand why she did not lose weight. She was ostensibly following my recommended regime, and on her own initiative was taking vast quantities of vitamins and minerals. When I asked her whether she ate chocolate, she told me emphatically that she had not eaten it for years. I was convinced she was not telling the truth and that beneath the very large bed from which she received me there was probably a chocoholic's paradise that she wallowed in when she was alone. Her staff later told me this was indeed the case. Neither I nor any other therapist could help her if she was not prepared to be honest.

Do not hesitate to 'baby' yourself. If it helps to count every time you chew a mouthful of food, do it. If reminders about volume or eating slowly keep you concentrated, use them. Be prepared to make up your own rules of self-persuasion as you go along. Whatever works for you cannot be wrong.

Is There Life After the Basic Programme?

Not in the way you have known it. Unfortunately, we cannot have our cake and eat it. The idea that as long as we do the occasional penance or undergo short-term corrective treatment we can do as we like in terms of how we live, and stay healthy, is a non-starter for all but the doughtiest constitutions. Future illness can only be avoided or its negative effects lessened if the Basic Programme is accepted as an ongoing regime. It is not a quick-fix designed to get us back to our 'normal' bad habits as soon as possible. I have much more energy now than I had twenty years ago, and that is simply due to the fact that I have learnt how to look after myself. We can all learn to work on our bodies and make them happier, and the more diligent we are the greater will be our health dividend. Any assistance you can give your system to make it less sluggish, less overloaded, will be repaid, especially later in life.

The rate at which your body responds to any of the programmes will depend on how well you follow the instructions and on your state of health. It takes us years to degrade the body and if we are some way down the degeneration road we cannot expect to restore it to something approaching a state of grace virtually overnight. If we want to get better and stay better, we have to learn to appreciate and keep faith with the small improvements in ourselves. The body can be turned around, in some extreme cases perhaps not completely, but we should not expect the process to be speedy or easy. If you have been constipated for many years, your progress will be slower than that of somebody who has not. The same applies if you have low blood sugar or have an unfavourable genetic inheritance relative to that of a friend or neighbour.

We cannot choose our bodies, and although some people may spend a great deal of time and money changing them cosmetically in ways that nature never intended, at some point we have to be content to live with what we have got. People tend to be totally taken up with appearances. These are what impress the imagination, and so vital parts are nipped and tucked or pulled and stretched to fit an ideal of beauty or style – usually someone else's. But in becoming like a tailor's dummy there is a danger of forgetting a basic truth: essentially, the most attractive element of any human being is not their looks but the inner energy they generate. Many years ago an ex-boyfriend of mine went off with another woman. I demanded to know what she looked like. He said: 'Oh, I can't remember her face because it wasn't her own'. By all accounts she was a woman who had the perfect nose, mouth, eyes and shape, but she was totally unmemorable as a human being.

The same reasoning applies to our blueprint. Accepting that we are different and that we are weak in some areas is not so difficult when we become more balanced. It is futile to ignore our particular 'cross', because it will not magic itself away. Our differences – physical, emotional, intellectual, spiritual – are what mark us out as individuals. Instead of disowning the bits we do not like about ourselves – and taking the 'Oh, she's with someone else' line – we should embrace them. Perhaps there is a higher reason for our characteristics, and hidden in them are valuable lessons we need to learn if we are to move on and develop.

The same applies to the people we meet and the relationships we form. We should try to remain open to learning throughout our lives, even when it comes from the most unlikely quarters – from our children, godchildren, grandchildren, nieces or nephews, the children of friends. Wisdom cannot be counted in years. Only by engaging with life on all levels will we find out who we really are and what we are capable of. This is, for me, the great challenge and joy in keeping healthy.

Chapter Four

TREATMENT PROGRAMMES

The purpose of this section is to show how many common health conditions arise and the self-help measures that can be taken to ameliorate their effects. Major conditions have been deliberately excluded on the grounds that it would be neither appropriate nor useful to offer guidance.

One of the problems with presenting specific programmes is that illnesses themselves are rarely specific – often there are as many differences in symptoms, constitution and personality as there are similarities. I take this into account when I treat a patient. You will have to learn what is right for you, and where your requirements differ from what is suggested. One good habit to get into is that of constantly monitoring yourself. You may find, for example, that one teaspoon of Cal-M suits you better than two teaspoons. That is as it should be. Many healing crises could be avoided if people were prepared to proceed carefully by testing their responses. Never follow instructions blindly. Trust the response of your own body. Each of us is different and our responses to foods and medicines will reflect that difference. Remember: you might be a flower for the desert not for the mountains. If you get a reaction such as a rash or a headache to something you are taking, leave it for a few days and then try it again but at a reduced dosage. Many people mistakenly think that a reaction is a sign of allergy or that it is a necessary part of treatment. Neither is the case. By reacting the body is telling you to proceed more slowly because it is not sure that it likes what you are doing. The treatment will receive a positive response when it decides that you are doing the right thing by it after all.

I never ask anyone to change what they are already doing in terms of taking medicines or purgatives. The body gets used to what it is given and it can be traumatizing when that something is suddenly withdrawn. Purgatives provide a classic example of this syndrome – the system can block if they are withdrawn abruptly. If you are on prescribed medication or are taking various vitamin and mineral supplements, there is no need to stop them while you follow the programmes. In the case of people who are receiving prescribed medicines, when the body is functioning better it will be up to your doctor to take the decision to alter or reduce medication.

As will be obvious from the programmes, I use organic supplements in preference to standard mineral and vitamin supplementation. The so-called Green Energy foods (see page 135) such as chlorella, spirulina or alfalfa or complete super-food products such as Missing Link (see page 138) contain the essential vitamins and minerals we need in easily absorbable forms. Most people find them easier to incorporate into a daily regime – one dose sprinkled on food daily instead of a range of tablets or capsules to be wound down.

In my practice I use various complex homeopathic preparations of different strengths for specific ailments. I have suggested Dr Reckeweg's preparations in some of the treatments included here. This is because of the complex formulas available they are, in my experience, the mildest and safest to use without professional supervision.

The rate at which the body responds to any of the treatments will depend on the starting point. If your fermentation is very poor and you have severe arthritis, you must expect progress to be slow. Generally it takes about eight weeks to start building up the bacterial flora, to adjust bad eating habits (volume, chewing, for example), to encourage the digestive enzymes and to even out blood sugar levels if these are a problem.

If you have several of the problems for which I have included treatments, prioritize. If you have headaches, get rid of the headaches before you worry about changing the bacterial flora. If you have wind or belching, tackle either first before you worry about losing weight. Do not concentrate on the wrong aspect. Assess how you are feeling within yourself rather than, for example, fretting about the fact that your spots are still in evidence. If you are beginning to feel more energetic and better within yourself, you are making progress. Once this corner has turned it will be only a matter of time before the spots disappear.

I have suggested additional remedies or therapies where I think they are appropriate. However, the basis of all the treatments is the diet. This must be changed if improvement is to be achieved. The priority in all of the treatments – and of this book – is the digestion. At the risk of boring you for the umpteenth time – if the fermentation and acidity of the gut are put right, you will start to absorb better and thus help your body generally, whatever your health problem.

ASTHMA

Asthma can develop at any time of life, although usually it appears in childhood and tends to run in families. Leading American nutritionist Dr Jonathan Wright attributes most cases of childhood asthma to low levels of acid in the stomach, enabling toxins to build up in the system. The individual's genetic make up means that these toxins will be channelled through the lungs. In most cases, there is a family history of weakness associated with the lungs, such as sinusitis, congestion or heavy colds. In older sufferers, osteoarthritis can develop. The pollution from car exhausts can trigger an attack of asthma, but more likely culprits are acid-forming foods, especially dairy products.

Asthmatics tend to love starch almost to the point of addiction and many of them believe that it poses less of a problem than cow's milk or cheese. Unfortunately, this is not the case – both bread and sugar can produce as speedy a reaction. All highly processed or refined foods, such as cakes, biscuits, ice cream, crisps, chocolates and sweets, must be eliminated from the diet. The preservative sulphur, found in, for example, most soft drinks, lager and dried apricots, can aggravate or provoke an attack of asthma. Salt, additives such as monosodium glutamate and food colourings should also be avoided.

Profile

Many asthmatics are worriers and strivers after perfection. They come across as tense, rather wound-up individuals because they tend to internalize their stress. So great can be their desire to please other people that rarely will they venture their own opinions for fear of being out of step with other people or causing offence.

Some of my asthma patients even worry about what their friends might say about the treatment. The prospect of being exposed to criticism for changing their diet terrifies them. I advise them to take the line of least resistance and avoid criticism, either by not telling their friends or by making an excuse as to why they cannot eat such a large lunch or a certain dish.

Treatment Plan

Use the Basic Programme as your basis (see page 55), and incorporate the following specific measures.

Immediately eliminate from the diet highly fermenting or acid-forming foods, such as sugar, sweets and wheat, and also foods that are mucous forming, such as dairy products. In some sufferers the problem with dairy products is so bad that all milk products must be eliminated, including those derived from goat's or sheep's milk, and soya products used instead. Nuts should be avoided, too, because they can have an irritating effect on an asthmatic digestive tract as they pass through the system, causing the gut to 'blow up'.

Poor digestion is common among asthma sufferers and it is often advisable for them to eat little and often so that food is not sitting in the system. In the afternoon a small bowl of chicken soup, half an avocado or grated apple gently cooked should blunt the desire for starch, such as crisps or sweet biscuits.

Constipation aggravates the problem and must be tackled. If it is present, more fibre, such as oatbran, should be taken with the fruit breakfast, or a few stewed prunes eaten in the evening (see page 75 for further advice).

It is important to eat proportionally more green leaf vegetables and fruit than protein. Remember the cupped hands and the ratio of foods these should contain: one third protein or starches, two-thirds vegetables and fruit.

Rice- or oat-based cereals should be substituted for wheat, which must be eliminated.

Take unsaturated oils such as safflower oil, sunflower oil, hempseed oil in capsule or liquid form and cod liver oil, which contains vitamins A and D, to help heal the lining of the respiratory tract. If you want to cook with oil, remember to use olive oil.

Infusions of sage or thyme (especially, because this will also shift the mucous on the chest) with honey are soothing, as are Mullein or a herbal tea containing liquorice.

Anything that reduces tension is of benefit. As its name suggests Cal-M is calming; it also feeds the liver and changes the acidity in the system gently (see page 127). For children, try half a teaspoon of Cal-M before they go to bed. If they do not like the taste, add it to a mug of soya milk or mix it with a little stewed apple and a drizzle of honey. Adults should take 2 level teaspoons of Cal-M.

Helping remedies

- Dr Reckeweg's homeopathic complex R 43.
- Relaxing essential oils such as eucalyptus, aniseed, sage and thyme are beneficial if used wisely. Do not forget to dilute them in a carrier or base oil, otherwise you may find yourself in a similar predicament to a patient of mine. He generously sprinkled neat essential oil into the bath, got in, felt a bit hot but thought no more about it until about half an hour later when, as he was driving along, his whole body blew up into blisters. His experience was extreme, because he was a diabetic and his skin was unusually dry and vulnerable. However, some essential oils can burn the skin of even healthy people and should be used with great care.

The Asthmatic Child

Children are more likely to become asthmatic if they have not had their mother's milk, which gives protection against a range of possible dangers, including cow's protein (see Milk, page 137). If a mother is not going to breast-feed, it is important that she chooses a baby food that is not based on cow's milk (goat's milk is an acceptable alternative) and that she aids the child's digestion with *Bifidobacterium infantis*. This will maintain the friendly flora in the gut. The gastrointestinal tracts of babies are sterile and as a result are open to colonization by harmful microorganisms. The beneficial Bifidobacterium is the principal intestinal bacteria in breast-fed infants and is present in far fewer numbers in bottle-fed babies.

It can be exceedingly difficult for a busy mother with a healthy child to provide a diet of balanced, interesting food. The dietary limitations that must be imposed by the mother of an asthmatic present a much greater problem. The trick is to change the diet around without the child noticing, by gradually introducing more vegetables, phasing out wheat-based products in favour of oat-based ones, and substituting honey for sugar.

Asthmatic children tend to yo-yo between bad skin and asthma. At any given time either one or the other will be active in getting rid of the overflow of toxins in the system; when the skin is bad the asthma will be all right, and vice versa. If the treatment plan is followed, the skin problems and the asthma should clear up simultaneously.

Helping Therapies

- Osteopathic adjustment of the vertebra linked to the lungs and lung function can bring relief. Acupuncture treatment can also improve breathing.
- Any gentle, calming, touching therapy, such as massage or reflexology, will help, especially to the back, stomach and feet.
- A rather more esoteric option is tuning, in which you learn to direct sound waves to all areas of the body. In one class I attended, people with sinus problems were streaming by the end of the session.
- Floatation therapy or body harmony in a float pool are wonderfully relaxing.
- Learning to breathe properly can be a revelation for many asthma sufferers. Yogic deep breathing techniques can be learnt but even people who have been doing yoga for years do not always perform these techniques properly; they may think they do, but in many cases they do not. It is possible to buy a machine that trains the breathing and provides feedback, thus avoiding the possibility of incorrect usage (see Breathing machine, page 126).

CATARRH / SINUSITIS

If they are experienced on a regular basis and not simply as the by-products of a cold, catarrh or sinusitis can be placed a few stops before asthma along the degeneration road. Both normally run in families. These conditions indicate an overflow via the lymphatic as the body eliminates what it cannot cope with. This is a healthy sign insofar as it shows the immune system is working properly. However, as with most stresses, there is another way.

Profile

Some people suffer with bad sinuses and that stuffy nose feeling all their lives. Most likely as children they were not robust, tending to appear pale and peaky. In my experience they like to eat sugary foods, especially ice ceam and milk products, because their digestion is not strong and these foods tend to slip down and not sit on them as do other foods. The problem with this diet, of course, is that it makes the system acid and creates the right conditions for infection by viruses.

Colds or flu, to my way of thinking, are a sign of toxins in the body. If the system was pure it would not fall prey to viral or bacterial infections. That said, life is life and most of us get a cold now and then. The most effective remedy for cold or flu symptoms is elderberry extract (see page 130). Cow's protein is a classic blocker of the lymphatic system and must be eliminated from the diet in order to clear out the sinuses and allow the system to regain energy.

Treatment Plan

Eliminate from the diet all products made with cow's milk.

Eliminate foods that ferment badly, such as wheat, and starchy and sugary foods.

Eat small volumes and chew thoroughly to ensure that all food is digested properly and so passes through the system rather than sitting there fermenting.

Until the catarrh clears or the sinuses unblock, eat cleansing foods, such as green vegetables and onions. Eat plenty of garlic too. As far as proteins are concerned, choose lighter types, such as fish and chicken.

To avoid a recurrence, follow the Basic Programme (see page 55), and keep your intake of cow's products to a minimum.

Helping Remedies

- Thyme, elderflower and mullein release the lymphatic and encourage the elimination of impurities. All can be taken in the form of an infusion or tea.
- Inhale eucalyptus, and any remedies including peppermint or lemon should be beneficial.
- Take echinacea (see page 130) to boost the immune system.

Helping Therapies

Try taking warm baths with soothing or antiseptic oils, such as lavender or tea tree.

CONSTIPATION

Constipation is normally a sign of low peptic acidity with no message from the stomach reaching the liver to trigger the release of bile. Bile is like washing-up liquid for the digestive system – a few squirts deal with the matter in the system. The aim of treatment is to get the liver to respond as it should to make the digestive system work properly. As well as being common among people who regard themselves as healthy, constipation is a frequent companion of many disorders, from diabetes to migraine, and if it continues for years can lead to serious bowel disease.

Few people like to admit to being constipated and prefer to put down the infrequency of their bowel movements to personal idiosyncrasy. Obviously there are degrees of constipation – a really constipated person is someone who goes to the toilet once a week. Constipation of that order causes headaches and muzziness. This is not surprising when you think about what is going on inside their digestive system. If food stays in the digestive system for longer than about two days it becomes acid and produces wind which causes pain. The longer it lies there the more putrid and toxic it becomes. The situation is not helped by the plentiful supplies of new matter which drop on top of the last delivery. And so the problem builds up, like a compost heap. Constipation leaves the body open to attack from those potentially destructive microflora you were reading about earlier (see page 17). The longer the intervals between bowel movements the more vulnerable the body is to negative microflora attack.

Profile

As usual we have to look ourselves for the answer to constipation. In my experience constipated people tend to be controllers. They find it difficult to let go, to take a back seat and let someone else do the running around. Because they insist on taking the helm and running the show, they are invariably worried and stressed by the burden they have heaped upon themselves. In a majority of cases, tension is the cause of constipation.

I have one perfect example of this for you. One patient of mine, who has been constipated for her entire life, was taken on a cruise by her husband. For the duration of that holiday, she was not constipated. As soon as she crossed the gangplank to disembark at the end of it, she was. I would describe this particular woman as a control freak and a perfectionist. While she was on holiday, her worries were someone else's and by switching off from them, she and her body were finally enabled to relax.

Interestingly, for many other people the reverse would probably have been the case. Think of the times you have been constipated on holiday. Anxiety induced in us by unfamiliar surroundings can be enough to block the system.

Treatment Plan

Constipation can take a long time to disappear from a sufferer's life, so bear this mind if you are about to follow the programme. If you are taking purgatives, continue with them. When the digestion improves, you will probably find that you do not need to take them as much or that a milder type, such as aloe vera or aniseed, is more appropriate. The long-term objective is for any type of purgative to be unnecessary.

Not surprisingly, the number one requirement is to learn to relax. Later on I suggest a few appropriate therapies, but only you can provide the principal help required. Look at your lifestyle – if you are always on the run, and have a 'routine' which is sacrosanct, stop and reassess. Make your well-being your priority – that means finding time to relax, and giving your digestion time to cope properly.

Each morning on waking drink a glass of water, then chew a green apple perfectly, then have another glass of water. The water flushes the system and the pectin in the skin of the apple prompts the liver to release more bile.

Constipated people tend to be bolters and shovellers – i.e. they eat a lot too quickly. Try a few tricks to put a brake on this tendency – use chopsticks or eat with a small fork or spoon.

If constipation is slight, try a blend of herbs and enzymes – Candistatin (see page 127) would be my recommendation – to detoxify the bowel.

Ways must be found of alerting the stomach to the fact that food is entering the system. Most constipated people are deficient in hydrochloric acid and pepsin. An aid which combines these two important protein-digesting enzymes can be taken to remedy this problem (see page 130). However, thorough chewing is as important. If food goes down in lumps, or the volume of the intake is too large, the enzymes will be fighting a losing battle.

Acid (as distinct from acid-forming) foods should be added to the diet to promote the secretion of digestive enzymes. Cider vinegar, lemon, beetroot (raw or taken in juice or capsule form) are examples of acid foods which break down protein and aid the digestion by ensuring that the right messages are sent. If the acid in the stomach is right the duodenum will get the message to release enzymes to further neutralize the partly digested matter it receives. This response will trigger the gall bladder, pancreas and liver to play their part in the digestive process. The most important of these in this context is the gall bladder – if the bile is flowing, protein will be digested and constipation cannot occur.

Lighten the load on the body by eating foods that your system will not find hard to digest, such as small quantities of white meat or fish with steamed or stir-fried vegetables. It is important for everybody to eat small amounts of protein, and for constipation-sufferers it is absolutely crucial. If we eat small amounts the body is at least capable of chemically sorting out what it receives. You could also try introducing some pre-digested or pre-fermented food into the diet, such as soya products or Umeboshi plums.

Fresh herbs can be chewed before eating, or bitter herbs taken with the meal itself. Herbs are wonderful natural digestive aids, especially mint, thyme, tarragon, rosemary and dill. Chewing a few leaves of one of these herbs will give the stomach the message it needs to start the digestive juices flowing.

Use Oligo-fibre complex (see Fibre on page 133) to help the body correct toxicity in the bowel.

Most very constipated people do not sleep well and tend to wake in the night. If this is happening it could be that you are eating too late and undigested food is regurgitating or causing discomfort. Eat earlier, and check that you are not overeating. If neither is the cause of your sleeplessness, see Insomnia on page 95 for further advice.

Helping Remedies

- Gentler, natural alternatives to proprietory purgatives (which tend to irritate the system) are lemon and ginger or lemon and olive oil (see the recipe on page 151), avocado, a tablespoon of aloe vera, beetroot or Sauerkraut juice before food, or a few prunes before bedtime. All will encourage a bowel movement. Do not try to force the pace by taking large amounts of them; a maximum of 3 tablespoons of the aloe vera, beetroot or Sauerkraut juice. The idea is to gradually move your system into a cycle where it does not need persuasion.

Helping Therapies

- Breathing exercises are an excellent way of making us more aware of our bodies. Highly stressed, constipated people rarely breathe properly, generally being too busy to be tuned into themselves in this way (see Breathing machine on page 126).
- Pilates (see page 139) gently exercise and strengthen the muscles, stimulating the whole body and thus the digestion.
- Cranial osteopathy is another good method of getting much needed energy into the system.
- Skin brushing helps to eliminate toxins by stimulating the circulation (see page 147).

CYSTITIS

Cystitis signifies that the urine is too acid and is irritating the lining of the bladder. If this whole area becomes inflamed the infection can affect the kidneys and cause even more problems and discomfort. In bad cases, where the infection has taken hold, antibiotics might be necessary. If this is so, the system should be built up after the course of antibiotics has been completed, by making it more alkaline and eliminating acid-forming foods.

Whatever action is taken to effect a change in another area of the body the kidneys will play a large part in the process. If changes are made in diet, for example, the kidneys automatically come under pressure. Losing weight often brings on a minor bout of cystitis because not enough water is being drunk and the acidity arising out of the lost pounds has irritated the bladder.

Profile

It has been said that cystitis can be brought on by a state of mind, a sense of no longer wanting to be a people pleaser. The following story supports this idea. I had a friend who agreed to spend Christmas in a cottage with a few girlfriends, all of whom were smokers and culinary incompetents. No sooner had she donned the apron and assessed the situation than she got cystitis. She ended up doing all the cooking and having to watch as the lion's share of the champagne she had brought with her – which, of course, she could not drink because of the cystitis – was consumed by a self-invited guest whom she disliked. She could not wait for the 'festivities' to end. When she got home she looked up cystitis in a book and was cheered by the explanation. Now that she was home, she no longer reminded herself of the 'pissed off' person of the description. She opened a bottle of champagne. The cystitis went.

Treatment Plan

This is very simple and consists principally of drinking as much water as possible (c. 4 litres/7 pints per day) to dilute the acidity and wash away the infection. You could add lemon or ginger, or both, to increase alkalinity and cleanse the system. Take this action as soon as the infection makes itself known. A kidney infection may develop if acid-forming food is being consumed, the bladder is inflamed and not enough water is being drunk so the urine is very concentrated.

Eliminate all acid-forming foods, especially bread and sugar, and substitute alkalizing foods (see page 61).

Anti-fungal foods such as garlic, fennel and aniseed will help clear up the infection.

Helping Therapies

- Relaxing therapies, such as water therapy, or those that direct the energy to where it is needed in the body, such as cranial osteopathy and reflexology, are especially beneficial.

FOOD POISONING

The people who get food poisoning are usually the ones with the weakest digestive systems; elderly people, for example, in whom hydrochloric acid in the stomach is usually lacking, are particularly vulnerable. If hydrochloric acid is present in sufficient amounts any nasty microorganisms do not get a chance to raise their ugly heads. An appropriately acidic stomach is like a vat in which all the contents are pickled into harmlessness and cannot cause problems when they move further along the system. Anyone who has food poisoning should look seriously at how they can aid their digestive system to make it work better. The first sensible precaution is to avoid foods that have given you problems in the past. The body has a memory and if you have once been poisoned by a food, it will remind you.

Profile

Everybody has been afflicted by 'traveller's tummy' at one time or another, but by and large it is avoidable. I can vividly recall a trip down the Nile. To a man, my fellow travellers succumbed to a particularly virulent stomach upset, the weakest going down first. I was not spared the same fate because my cabin door had been mysteriously marked. During the hiatus before the storm, I had been careful to help my digestion by eating sparingly and taking pickled limes and lemons with my food, whereas the others had ignored these natural cleansers and piled into three courses at breakfast, lunch and dinner.

Treatment Plan

The classic 'stoppers' are bitters, such as Underberg, Po Chi pellets and Fernet Branca. (Underberg and Fernet Branca can be found in most good supermarkets and off licences; Po Chi pellets can be obtained from any Chinese supermarket.)

Timing is very important with bitters. They are best taken as soon as you sense that trouble is brewing and can feel your digestion going awry and before the 'poisoning' develops into sickness and diarrhoea. If taken at this point, they will stop the fermentation in the stomach. If you are already feeling nauseous, they will encourage the body to eliminate whatever is festering and cause vomiting and diarrhoea. This will certainly clear your system but leave you feeling like a rag doll.

If the sickness and diarrhoea are accompanied by wind, take charcoal tablets.

On the diet front, restrict yourself to liquids, such as chicken or vegetable stock, or, if you have diarrhoea and are not nauseous, boiled rice. These will nourish you – and, in the case of the rice, will calm the stomach – while imposing no extra strain on your system, which cannot be expected to cope with the poisoning and the processing of food. Toast, that old standby for upset stomachs, is especially inappropriate and will encourage fermentation.

When you are over the worst and feel you can manage solids, start with small portions of light foods, such as chicken soup, steamed vegetables or stewed apple.

GOUT

Most people experience gout as severe needle-like pain in the joints, especially the big toe. The gout is the uric acid the liver could not cope with settling in the system. Interestingly, most female gout sufferers will not refer to their condition as gout but high uric acidity. Perhaps this owes a lot to the image of gout as a greedy or dissolute person's affliction.

Profile

Most gout sufferers have a build-up of undigested protein in their gut from years of eating too much protein, usually meat. Typically, they are slightly over-weight, although not in all cases – some sufferers are as as thin as reeds. The usual scenario for a gout attack is a holiday, when the pressure of work – which for most gout sufferers is intense – has temporarily been lifted and the adrenaline has stopped pumping.

Treatment Plan

Gout is not something that happens overnight, and it can certainly not be eliminated overnight. Treatment is aimed at unloading the liver and changing the bacterial flora, but slowly – cleaning up the system too quickly can make the situation worse.

The following treatment should be followed for three to four months. If the gout does not make itself felt again when the body is stressed, you will know the treatment has worked. A long-haul flight is a good test. If the physiological stresses and strains incurred by lack of clean air and having to sit still for hours on end can be borne without the gout reminding you of its existence, you are better.

Switch to lighter types of protein – for example, chicken and fish instead of large steaks or platefuls of roast beef or pork.

Eliminate seafood, which is very difficult to digest.

Strictly monitor the volume you eat – remember the two cupped hands rule (see page 31).

Eliminate heavy alcoholic drinks, such as spirits and port wine.

Take a mild (suitable for a child) model Acidophilus (see page 139) to help change the bacterial flora.

Incorporate into your diet unsaturated oils, such as Udo's oil (see page 144), which are rich in essential fatty acids, to clean the liver and pick up the toxins in the system.

Take the complex called Boswellia (see page 126).

Take Cal-M (see page 127) to ensure that you start absorbing trace elements.

Take Missing Link (see page 138).

Ensure that you drink 2–3 litres (3½–5 pints) of water per day. Tea or coffee do not count as substitutes. Try to find acceptable alternatives, such as herb teas or green tea. If none of these appeals, experiment. Try a dash of lemon with ginger and honey in boiling water. If you find still water unappetizing, fill two thirds of the glass with still water and the remaining third with carbonated water. Try water with a dash of fruit juice. You must ensure that you flush from your system the toxins that are gradually released during the cleaning up process.

Helping Therapies

- Vigorous exercise makes gout worse but a daily routine of gentle bodywork, such as swimming or Pilates, is beneficial. Reflexology and massage are helpful too.

HAEMORRHOIDS

Haemorrhoids, or piles, are literally varicose veins at the end of the digestive tract. They occur when the veins at this lower end of the colon, called the haemorrhoidal veins, become enlarged and often inflamed. Piles serve as a very good example of what acidity means as far as the body is concerned. In short, acidity, caused by undigested proteins and sugars, makes the body swell. Alkalinity has the reverse effect.

Profile

Haemorrhoids are the Number One secret illness. They are rarely talked about and yet for many people are ever-present. I regard piles as I do ulcers; both stem from the same source – undigested protein which has fermented for a long time and become increasingly acid. Few people, it seems, make the connection between them and the digestion. Piles sufferers are usually sedentary types who eat more protein than is good for them. In many cases there is not enough acid in the stomach to cope with the volume of food. This causes the system to become congested and the person constipated. The surest cure is to stop over-indulging in red meat and highly refined foods.

Treatment Plan

Ironically, piles can put in an unwelcome appearance if the change to a better diet is made too quickly. The haemorrhoids can easily be aggravated and possibly be made to bleed if the toxic contents of the colon are stirred up too quickly. The challenge is to redress the balance in the system so that it becomes more alkaline without making the piles worse. This means proceeding slowly and with care.

Pay particular attention to the volume of each meal. The problem will be perpetuated if large quantities of food continue to be ingested and add to the existing toxic debris.

Eliminate all acid-forming foods (see page 62). The diet should consist largely of foods that will promote an alkaline ash, such as steamed or stir-fried vegetables, rice, and avocados (see page 62).

One or two salted, pickled Umeboshi plums eaten each day will also help to change the acidity, reduce the inflammation and encourage the haemorrhoids to heal.

A fibre which does not provoke too much wind, thereby aggravating the piles, is advisable for the constipation; also see the treatment for constipation on page 75.

Take Cal-M (see page 127) on food.

Helping Remedies

- Try Dr Reckeweg's R42 homeopathic remedy.

- Homeopathic suppositories, such as Anisan (made by the German company Pascoe), are especially helpful; these make the veins contract and heal the affected area.

Helping Therapies

- Any therapy that gently energizes the system and makes it less sluggish is beneficial, such as reflexology, swimming or water therapy.

HEADACHE

If you ask most people why they get headaches, most will say either that they do not know or that they had too many drinks the night before. The 'Don't knows' will look round for reasons, and might settle on the weather as a factor (perhaps it is an overcast, thundery day) or that they have held one position for too long and made themselves stiff, for example by working at a PC. No one will consider that what they have eaten, or not eaten, could be responsible.

Food can have precisely the same effect as alcohol when it comes to upsetting the liver. The unlikely chemical changes that food can bring about in the body is evidenced by the following story. A Mormon was stopped by traffic police in Utah and subsequently prosecuted for driving while under the influence of drink. It turned out that the diet of this very large man – who was, needless to say, strictly teetotal – consisted almost entirely of sugared blueberry muffins. He was like a walking distillery and had made the alcohol in his own system.

Profile

People with a tendency towards headaches are usually constipated and overloading the liver via the gut. They eat too quickly and often are low blood sugar types (see page 102); a drop in the blood sugar level, probably because they have not eaten, is enough to bring on a headache in them. Sometimes sufferers will experience a feeling of the digestion being out of sorts before the headache comes on.

However, the question any headache sufferer should ask themselves is why is the liver under pressure? Headache is the spillover that the liver could not take. If you ask yourself what you have done, the straw that broke the camel's back will in most cases float into your mind. Look back over the preceding three days –

Did you eat lots of cheese, chocolate or orange? All three are classic headache-inducers. If you love chocolate, eat real chocolate, not the excuse for it that makes up the bulk of confectionery stocks in most shops and supermarkets; these horrors are mostly composed of fats and sugar. One or two very small knobs of an 80 per cent dark chocolate should not do any harm – but wait until you are better and the liver is no longer under pressure.

Did you drink enough water? Remember the one and a half to two litre (two and a half to three and a half pint) rule – drinking alcohol would have exacerbated any shortfall.

Did you have more coffee than usual?

If you can discover what caused your headache, you will avoid repeating the same mistake in future.

Treatment Plan

Headache indicates a slight toxic overload of the system, and that the liver is under pressure via the gut. When people come to me with a string of problems which includes headache, that is usually the first thing to get better once the system begins to clean up. Cleaning up the system too quickly can actually cause a headache, even in someone who has not had a headache before.

Follow the Basic Programme (see page 55), incorporating these modifications:

If you are constipated, follow the programme on page 75.

Eliminate all wheat products.

Eliminate all cow's protein and chocolate from your diet.

Cut down on coffee gradually – stopping suddenly might actually bring on a headache.

Eat little and often. Reduce the volume of meals – remember the hands rule, see page 31. Take chicken or vegetable stock mid-morning or mid-afternoon to keep the blood sugar even.

Increase the intake of water between meals (2–3 litres/3½–5 pints daily).

Add trace elements to the diet by taking Cal-M (see page 127) at night.

Aid the digestion with herbs such as Feverfew (see page 133) and digestive enzymes (see page 130).

Have warming drinks of Chinese or Japanese green tea, fennel, or lemon and ginger.

Helping Therapies

- Cranial osteopathy is excellent for headache sufferers because it helps the flow of energy. Massaging the neck muscles helps, as do relaxing, warm baths. The worst effects of a headache can be offset by drinking a lot of water, relaxing or going for a walk. (See also Migraine, page 111)

HIGH BLOOD PRESSURE

The person with high blood pressure, or hypertension, has usually been pushing their body hard for a long time and habitually drawing on adrenaline to maintain their impetus and motivation. In most sufferers the body has already sent out distress signals – such as diarrhoea or constipation, excess weight and high cholesterol – which have been ignored. Forcing the body on causes the insulin level to run high all the time and thus the blood pressure. Raising the blood pressure increases the amount of glucose in the blood and narrows the smaller blood vessels.

Profile

The high blood pressure person feels more or less as any individual would who has drunk five pints of coffee in quick succession – irritable. It does not take much for them to become very angry or agitated – a car in front of theirs travelling too slowly or blocking their way is often enough to make them lose their temper. The constant high revving during daylight hours is also felt when the body should be calm and at rest – people with high blood pressure usually do not sleep well. In both men and women the main underlying feature of high blood pressure is the same: worry, even if in some instances there may seem to be very little for them to worry about. Some people can worry about changing the curtains or taking the car to the garage. This is not to trivialize. Perception is all and what one person may regard as insignificant another will consider a major problem. The point is how each individual reacts in a given set of circumstances. Unfortunately, the person with high blood pressure reacts in a way that undermines their health.

There is a close link between high blood pressure and low blood sugar (see page 102). Many low blood sugar people go on to develop high blood pressure.

High blood pressure is rare in the young, tending to come later in life when the body has been drained of its flexibility. The tendency for the condition to run in families may be explained by the notion of learnt behaviour; for example, if a parent is always shuffling their feet, looking at their watch or darkly muttering 'Come on' while waiting for a bus, their child is likely to follow that example and replicate the pattern.

Treatment Plan

Reducing high blood pressure involves using the Basic Programme as the basis (see page 55) and looking at ways of slowing the body so that it can find a more natural, less hectic rhythm. For many people with high blood pressure, however, it is simply not feasible for them to slow down as much as they should. What people in this situation can do is to help themselves by taking foods that are easy to digest and that keep their energy more even – such as alfalfa – and avoiding those – such as gingseng – that will race the body even more.

High blood pressure people tend to eat too much very quickly. Some might eat one big meal a day, usually in the evening, in the mistaken belief that by missing out on breakfast (apart from a cup of coffee) and lunch they are slimming. Therefore, the first points to look at are:

1. Volume – gradually reduce this. If it is done too quickly there is a risk of getting super-hungry and bingeing on chocolate bars and other simple carbohydrates.
2. Do not miss meals – ensure that breakfast, lunch and dinner are eaten.
3. Eat slowly and in a relaxed manner.

These three measures are essential for good digestion. If the digestive system can be made to work properly the blood pressure level will reduce.

As far as the diet itself is concerned, all foods or substances that stimulate and get the adrenaline pumping should be eliminated, specifically:

Coffee and traditional Indian tea.

Short, quick-lift drinks and foods, such as soft drinks, crisps, biscuits and sweets.

Salt – a high intake of sodium has been linked to high blood pressure and must be avoided.

Red meat and pork – these heavy meats leave an acid ash deposit that builds up in the arteries, especially if they are eaten in large quantities.

Alcohol should be taken in moderation. If a small glass of scotch or wine helps you to unwind in the evening, then by all means have it. The only habit you need to break is that of over-consumption or dependence. Alcohol is a problem if you must have it as soon as you get home after work.

If you are a smoker, try to cut down.

Take Missing Link (see page 138) – this helps to reduce the levels of both cholesterol and blood pressure.

Take Udo's oil (see page 144) – this picks up sticky, undigested plaque in the system.

If you get headaches while the fermentation in the gut is changing, drink more water and proceed more slowly.

Helping Remedies

- If symptoms of stress or anxiety are acute, take Cal-M (see page 127) throughout the day; if they are not, take it at night to feed the liver. Hypericum (St John's Wort) or Bach's Rescue Remedy will also help in calming the system.

Helping Therapies

- Anything that makes life less of a drama or worry and more fun should reduce high blood pressure. It could be sitting sniffing roses, going for a walk, swimming, or going to a therapist to receive massage, shiatsu or reflexology treatment. It is especially important that the therapy does not create more tension than it dissipates. I have known people with high blood pressure to become so irritated with some forms of therapy that their whole treatment – including my part in it – has been blocked. Find a therapy that does not have this effect. Do not be swayed by other people when making your choice.

Decide on the basis of what appeals to you. If you find that the therapy you have chosen is not appropriate after all, try something else. When patients with high blood pressure are happy with a therapy they respond very well and quickly get in touch with themselves.

Note: If you are taking medication prescribed by your doctor, do not stop taking it. When your body is functioning better and the blood pressure is reducing, your doctor will be the one who decides to alter or reduce your medication.

HIGH CHOLESTEROL

High cholesterol indicates to me a liver under pressure in a person who is not digesting protein well. Cholesterol is a substance widely distributed throughout the body which is synthesized principally by the liver. It is essential for the production of the sex hormones, as well as the repair of membranes. Cholesterol also makes up a large part of the fatty deposits that may block the blood vessels in the life-threatening condition known as atherosclerosis. Unless you have a major genetic problem or an exceptionally bad diet (of which more below), high cholesterol is unlikely to crop up before the age of 35.

Profile

Normally the high cholesterol type person is acidic as a result of large amounts of undigested food in the system. The tendency is for them to eat too much and to be constipated. I think of high cholesterol people as the cousins of the high blood pressure type (see page 86) – that is, tending to be impatient, quick tempered, fast eaters and stressed. High blood pressure and high cholesterol often go together, but not always. Overweight and high cholesterol do not automatically go together either.

One man in his mid-thirties came to me and said, 'I went to my doctor and I have high cholesterol, but, really, look at me, I'm slim.' I asked him what he ate. He replied, 'That's just it. I only eat chocolate biscuits and crisps'. He did not believe that he could have high cholesterol because he was so slim. This is a myth that needs exploding. Biscuits and crisps are almost entirely composed of saturated fats and sugars, the very foods that raise the cholesterol level. The fact that he was pencil slim was an irrelevance. He did not eat enough volume to get fat but his body was living on foods that were not nourishing it. He felt hungry much of the time and yet if he tried to eat more than a small amount he felt peculiar.

His aversion to eating was based on practicality – he did not have time to sit down to eat a proper meal, let alone prepare one himself, and eating the fast foods of his choice met his energy requirements. Fortunately, the shock of being told he had high cholesterol persuaded him to make time and change his diet. Now, he is eating properly at defined meal times.

It is not difficult to raise the cholesterol level by just a few days of eating unwisely. A high-powered businessman with a very bad digestive system who had been coming to me for some time went off to Brussels. When he set off his digestion was right, the acidity in his system was balanced, he had lost weight and he was generally in good shape. He returned home feeling below par and immediately went to his doctor, who checked him over and told him his cholesterol was raised. The man telephoned me and said, 'All this treatment has given me high cholesterol. What have you done?'.

I said that I had not given him anything that would raise his cholesterol level and that the diet I had put him on would not have had that effect either. I asked him to give me some time to think about what could possibly have gone wrong. He rang off, still convinced that it must be my fault. I rang him back later and asked him a few questions about the days he had spent away. Had he done anything special? I knew he had been in Brussels on his own, without his family. He said 'No'. When I suggested a few possibilities, such as enjoying the night life or eating something unusual, he said, 'Oh no, except that I had a pint of Häagen-Dazs ice cream every night before I went to bed'. He was very surprised when I told him that this innocent nocturnal pleasure was the cause of the problem.

Treatment Plan

The cholesterol level will right itself if the gut is working well and is properly nourished. The treatment is aimed at clearing away the undigested proteins in the system. Follow the Basic Programme on page 55, incorporating the following adjustments.

Eliminate proteins that are hard to digest, such as red meat, (beef, pork, etc.), processed meat, such as sausages, seafood (mussels, lobster, etc.), and cheese. Eat white meat (poultry and game birds) and fish, especially oily types, such as mackerel and sardines, which are high in omega-3 essential fatty acids (see page 131) and will help reduce the level of cholesterol in the blood. Unsaturated omega-6 rich oils such as linseed, safflower and hemp also have this effect.

Reduce your intake of stimulants, such as coffee, tea and alcohol. Instead drink water and herbal teas.

Take the whole lemon and olive oil drink (see page 151) daily.

Take Missing Link (see page 139).

Take olive leaf tincture.

Helping Remedies

- Any remedy that aids the liver should be beneficial. Try milk thistle (see page 137).
- Take Cal-M (see page 127) at night. In cases of high cholesterol the liver is often short of magnesium and Cal-M will rectify this deficiency.
- To help dissolve the cholesterol, ensure that fennel and garlic – two excellent system cleansers – are included in the diet.

Helping Therapies

- The advice given under the treatment for high blood pressure (see page 86) about the importance of finding a therapy that makes you feel happy also applies here. A therapy that you are not comfortable with or has the effect of putting you in a bad frame of mind will do you no good, whatever the wonderful benefits it has been shown to bring to other people with high cholesterol.
- Oxygen therapy, also known as chelation (see page 129), is particularly appropriate for high cholesterol because it clears the veins of clogging debris and so removes much of the worry patients have about suffering a stroke or a heart attack.

IMPOTENCE

Impotence in men is not unlike PMS in women. Both show that the body needs to clear up and lighten the load on the liver. When the body is clear, sexual energy is not normally absent. If impotence is a problem, the first question that needs to be asked is: 'Why is my body in such a state it cannot function properly?' Adding testosterone is certainly not the answer. Just like every other part of the physiological jigsaw puzzle the sexual organs are affected by the overall health of the body. If the body is using its energies elsewhere, perhaps to keep us going at a high performance rate for twelve hours or more each day, there will not be much, if any, spare for sex. In major illness, such as diabetes, the sex drive diminishes very early. In a few patients I have inadvertently caused temporary impotence by clearing the liver too quickly – the relief on their faces when, having plucked up the courage to tell me about this new problem, they learn that it has been my fault and is not a reflection on their manhood.

Profile

Often with my patients I will discover that impotence has been a problem only when they are on the mend. One man who had come to me overweight and feeling depressed confided once his digestion was better: 'I think it's now working a bit below too'. At the age of 75 he probably felt a bit sheepish about mentioning it at all. His was a straightforward case of someone whose energy was low and once this had been regained several problems were solved simultaneously, including the sexual. The emotional and psychological dimensions of impotence are to my mind, however, more significant, and as a result sometimes more intractable.

The amount of sexual energy we possess is determined by our life force. This life force does not necessarily dim with age. If it is nurtured properly, it can strengthen with the passing years and burn more brightly. In too many cases, however, it becomes like the body it inhabits, sluggish and its appetite blunted. One reason for this can be found in the nature of modern relationships and the pressure imposed on them by our performance-oriented culture. Men and women have to be seen to measure up to an arbitrary modish ideal that takes no account of them as individuals. This can be particularly destructive to men, because once the designer suit has been shed they can so obviously be seen to fail.

This situation would not be so common if men stopped regarding sex as a push-button affair. Unfortunately, many of them are stuck in a time warp of their own making. The nature of sexual energy changes as we age, and woe betide the man who does not realize when he has passed from one phase to the next. According to an old man of my acquaintance, there are three principal phases. In the first, teenage, phase the young man is potent with all sexual partners, his willy like a magic lamp which has only to be gently rubbed for a few moments to glow with energy and desire. In the second, maturation, phase, he has to like his sexual partners. In the third, mature, phase he has to love them. Some men are so fixated on the physical mechanics of sex that they do not realize this development is taking place at a deeper level. They want to remain in that teenage, push-button phase forever, and when they are persistently denied it by their bodies, they become increasingly stressed.

If people have joy in their lives, sex is not a problem. It becomes a chore, as indeed do most things in life, if we make a routine of it or we are unhappy in the relationship. Life is constantly moving on and we should not be afraid to move with it. There has to be growth in a relationship for people to remain genuinely interested in each other. There has to be air between them, outside hobbies or pursuits, other friends. Too often in relationships frustration and claustrophobia succeed in debasing sex to the level where it becomes a crude bargaining counter in a destructive game instead of a gift shared by mutually loving individuals. Nor should one side of a relationship be expected to do all the loving and understanding and remain happy and contented. Both male and female energies need to be topped up by a turn basking in the warmth and attention of the other's love. If each of us receives our fair share of love, usually we will shine back beautifully.

Treatment Plan

Healthy people with efficiently functioning digestions are not as a rule lacking in sexual energy. In my experience there is always a larger problem lurking behind impotence, and it is this larger problem that needs to be identified. Unfortunately, the almost universal male fixation on the least significant few inches of their anatomy leads many sufferers to waste their time and money on aphrodisiacs instead of addressing the real problem. Sufferers need to look at the overall lack of vitality in the body and discover its source. Is there an ongoing, known weakness, such as high cholesterol, raised blood pressure, migraine or asthma? When you have identified the problem, turn to the appropriate programme.

INDIGESTION

Indigestion signifies that the digestive juices are not flowing as they should. There are two reasons for this: eating the wrong food, and tension. In some indigestion sufferers the two causes coincide. Indigestion can be an early staging post along the route to major disorders such as diverticulitis and ulcer, so the wise person will try to nip it in the bud as early as possible.

The aim of the treatment is to heal the stomach lining, and this means eliminating foods that are likely to discomfort the digestion, such as those that are acid-forming and fatty. Whichever cause the indigestion can be attributed to, follow the programme below for at least two weeks. The schedule is quite strict and must be adhered to if the lining is to heal.

Treatment Plan

Always sit down to eat. If you have got into the habit of eating on the move, perhaps snatching a sandwich between appointments or while you shop at lunchtime, break the habit. Allow at least fifteen minutes to elapse between eating your food and getting on with any tasks. The body cannot cope with you rushing and the process of digestion.

Make sure you are calm when you eat, and do not hurry. For example, while you are eating, do not agitate yourself by dwelling on the thousand and one tasks waiting for you. Try to think of eating time as your time. Ring fence it in your mind.

Chew your food very thoroughly to ensure that none of the matter scratches the digestive tract as it goes down. It is very easy to forget that what we eat can literally inflict wounds internally, and a stomach prone to indigestion is very tender.

Eliminate nuts and all fermenting or acid-forming foods (see page 62). Rice, rice pasta, millet and quinoa (taken in small amounts) are the only acceptable starches. The diet should consist of vegetables – steamed or cooked gently in stock and herbs (this Japanese method of cooking vegetables is easier on the digestion than stir-frying in oil) – with small quantities of light protein, such as fish (not shellfish) and meat. Avoid eating raw vegetables or salad until the lining has healed.

Take L-Glutamine (see page 134) to heal the lining of the stomach.

INSOMNIA

Insomnia can be physical or emotional in origin or a combination of the two. Both types offer interesting examples of how our two brains – the one in the head and the one in the gut – communicate and react off each other – and did we but know, probably exchange a few uncomplimentary gurgles about how we mistreat them. In many people insomnia occurs when the food they have eaten during the day sits in their system fermenting, causing discomfort and provoking enough worry to prevent them sleeping. If you are prone to this type of insomnia, look at ways to improve how you digest your food during the day. Similarly, if you make a habit of missing meals, causing your blood sugar to yo-yo, your body will become stressed and force you to pay the price in sleeplessness.

If bad eating habits are hindering absorption, the body will use whatever is at its disposal to make up the shortfall. The loss of daylight triggers the release in the gut of an amino acid that should travel to the brain and tell it that it is time to wind down for sleep. In someone who is short on nutrition, this amino acid will be gobbled up en route and so the message will not reach its destination.

In people who are prone to anxiety, sleeplessness is usually caused by the worry of the day carrying on into the night. A calm problem-free day leaves no such trace to trouble the senses. If insomnia is not to become a habit, one has to look at ways of controlling the anxiety. The most obvious way is to put into perspective whatever is troubling you, either by thinking it through in your own mind or by talking about it to someone who can be relied upon to be constructive. Be careful about whose ear you bend with your woes. If you are feeling like Job there is little point in discussing your situation with someone who will reinforce your negativity.

If the insomnia is total and has built up over weeks or months of strain, it is essential to feed the liver as well as calm the system and dissipate the tiredness. This cannot be achieved without input from the patient, who must be prepared to explore ways of reducing the burden they are placing on themselves. Slowing down and making time is often a problem for people, but essential if a breakdown or more serious illness is to be avoided.

Treatment Plan

There are two stages in the treatment for insomnia. The first part is to improve the digestion. If the gut is made to function better, a better sleeping pattern will result. Look at the Basic Programme on page 55 for guidance on how to improve your eating habits and the body's ability to absorb the nutrients it needs.

If you are taking medication, such as sleeping pills, do not suddenly stop taking them. Tail them back slowly after you have changed your diet and you have begun to feel better in yourself. Self-assessment is critical. Monitor your progress as you continue with the diet and experiment with the second-stage suggestions given below.

Avoid stimulants such as coffee and chocolate.

Calcium added to any warm drink has a calming effect. Try Cal-M (see page 127), which is a combination of calcium and magnesium; a lack of magnesium can cause early waking and unrefreshing sleep. Sip it throughout the day to keep the liver and the nervous system fed.

Re-focus your mind away from your worries, perhaps by reading or doing some gentle yoga stretching exercises. Meditating on one's own breath is a wonderfully calming technique although not practicable for someone who is very tense and anxious.

Sprinkle sea salt (Dead Sea salts are the strongest) or Epsom salts into a bathtub of warm water. The salt drains toxins from the system, leaving the body feeling heavy and ready for sleep.

Eat something light before you go to bed, such as stewed apple or prunes, to calm the system and feed the liver.

Take a warm drink before bedtime, such as malted milk or barley cup (preferably one with no or very little sugar in it). If milk makes you thick-throated, try calming herbal teas, such as vervain or chamomile.

Helping Remedies

- Try a homeopathic or herbal sleep-inducer, such as valerian, verbena, kava-kava or crateagus. You may have to experiment to find one that suits you; valerian, for example, is known to give some people bad dreams.

IRRITABLE BOWEL SYNDROME

Irritable bowel syndrome is usually found in people who have spent their entire lives constipated and in whom the fermentation has irritated the gut wall, causing diarrhoea as the body tries to expel the irritant.

Profile

Unless you have been on antibiotics for a long time or on a very high starch diet, irritable bowel is unlikely to develop before the age of about 45. The sort of people who tend to get irritable bowel usually eat too much starch and do not digest it properly because of bad eating habits. They tend to be worriers who miss meals and who put all their tension on their stomach when they do eat. In this situation the stomach does not produce any digestive enzymes, no message is sent to the liver or pancreas and so undigested food sits in the system and festers. Most men who show signs of developing irritable bowel tend to plough on regardless, masking their discomfort with indigestion pills and discounting the idea that it could be anything serious. Among women sufferers, irritable bowel tends to occur to people who have been on protein diets. These diets clog the body with undigested protein matter, making the gut wall sticky and the system constipated.

One step on from irritable bowel syndrome is colitis, and another step farther than that diverticulitis, in which the gut wall sags into small pockets where undigested matter becomes trapped and causes inflammation. The treatment for all three conditions is the same.

Treatment Plan

The road to recovery from diverticulitis is marked by very boring, bland food. Starches, raw vegetables and most fruit are among the most difficult foods for sufferers to digest. All vegetables must be baked or well steamed; even crisp vegetables must not be taken initially. Oil can irritate the system as can fresh herbs that are not chewed well or slightly cooked. It is especially important in the acute stages for liquids to be warm; this will help the stomach relax. Cold liquids can be a shock to the stomach and make it 'blow up'.

The importance of getting the basics of sensible eating absolutely right – i.e. paying attention to the volume of each meal and thorough chewing – cannot be over-emphasized in cases of irritable bowel or diverticulitis.

Treatment has to be taken in stages. The first step is to calm the system.

Weeks One and Two

Avoid starches, raw vegetables and fruit (papaya and stewed fruit excepted).

Exclude all acid-forming food, such as, pasta, bread, pulses and red meat, and those that tend to grate on the digestive tract, such as nuts.

Take small main meals of fish or chicken with cooked vegetables every 3–4 hours.

Take a mild digestive enzyme, such as Bio-Care's Enzyme Aid (see page 131).

Eat fresh herbs such as dill and fennel with your food to aid digestion.

Week Three

The digestion should be calming down, with less bloating and wind. Continue with the regime for weeks one and two. Introduce a weak (suitable for a child) milk-free model of Acidophilus (see page 124).

Week Four

The next stage is to heal the gut. You will know that you are ready for this phase of the treatment when the system is less windy and your energy is more constant.

Continue to eat carefully, following the regime given above.

Continue with the Acidophilus.

Sip L-Glutamine (see page 134) in water during the day.

To assist bowel movements, take fibre (for example Fructo-lite) on your food (see page 133). This may give more wind initially. Work up slowly, taking half a teaspoon at the start and gradually increasing the dosage to one teaspoon. You may need to reduce the dosage if your system objects by producing excessive wind.

Week Five

You are ready for this stage if the stool is getting softer, and the bloatedness, wind and energy are continuing to show improvement.

Continue to eat carefully, but start to introduce a wider range of proteins. If you are a meat-eater, this could include grilled red meat.

Introduce lemon and olive oil into the diet. You can take this either in drink form (see page 151 for recipe), made up into a sauce (which is easier to take if the system is very delicate, because it does not burn so much) or put directly onto the food.

Take Missing Link (see page 138) to keep the blood sugar even.

Continue with the L-Glutamine, possibly tailing back the dosage if bowel movements are daily and improvement is marked.

Continue with the fibre.

Change to a slightly stronger model Acidophilus – my recommendatation would be Bio-Acidophilus, a combination of *Lactobacillus acidophilus* and Bifidobacterium. Alternatively, ask for advice at the healthfood store or chemist where you purchased the first model.

Week Six

Continue to eat carefully but start to add more variety to the diet, including raw foods. Try small amounts of avocado, spinach or endive and more herbs. However, avoid raw foods that are likely to make the stomach blow up, such as tomato and lettuce.

Try eating some sourdough bread, chewed very well. Monitor how well you digest this and your other food. If you have signs of bloating and windiness, you will know you are progressing too quickly and need to retrace your steps.

Continue with the Acidophilus and the Missing Link.

Helping Remedies

- Dr Reckeweg's homeopathic complex R5 will reduce the sensation of bloatedness in the stomach.
- The bitter herb angelica (see page 125) is an effective reliever of wind.
- Fennel, sage, peppermint or chamomile herbal teas will calm and aid the digestion.

Helping Therapies

- Any therapy that calms the digestive system and stops it 'revving' will help, such as reflexology, massage, acupuncture, aromatherapy, body balancing in salt water or shiatsu.

The Aftermath

If you have once had irritable bowel syndrome, colitis or diverticulitis, you must accept the fact that you will never be able to eat exactly what you please without risking a flare up. Even when the system has healed, you will need to be careful and to eat all foods, but especially proteins, in moderation.

- Exclude all spicy foods, such as curry and chilli con carne permanently.
- Exclude all types of nuts permanently.
- Be very wary of all products containing gluten. However, even this 'problem' agent can be transformed by the pre-digestion that occurs when we chew our food to perfection.

Bloatedness and belching wind are signs that the system is coming under pressure again. If they appear, start to tidy up by returning to the regime outlined above.

JOINT PROBLEMS

All joint problems, such as arthritis, are produced by acidity in the body. This acidity can be caused by high intakes of antibiotics or sugar, or incompletely digested food. The bacteria that grow in the bowel as a result of incomplete digestion cause inflammation of the synovial membrane lining the bones at joints and covering many tendons. Dairy products, such as milk and eggs, can cause joint pain in some people. Unless one is extremely aware the body becomes progressively more toxic with age because of the slow-down in its production of digestive enzymes. There are few people aged 80 who have not got at least a slight build up of acidity in their joints.

Rheumatism, too, has acidity at its root, as do frozen shoulder, tennis elbow, lumbago or back pain. Over-exercising produces an excess of lactic acid in the joint which can take a long time to clear. The problem with this type of injury is that it occurs inside the ligaments and cannot be healed directly via the lymphatic system. If you start to get stiff when playing a sport or working out, do not exercise through it in the hope that the stiffness will wear off. Over-use of any part of the body necessitates a re-balancing and a return to alkalinity.

The older the person with joint problems is the harder he or she has to work. Attitude, though, is nine-tenths of the battle and if the desire for change is there, gradually and with patience an improvement will come about. The patient must learn to feel his or her way, talk to the body and listen to it.

Profile

One of the worst cases of arthritis I have treated was a woman in her mid-forties. She approached me because she had been on anti-inflammatory drugs for about five years to keep the arthritis under control and these were now making her feel ill. She was a highly stressed type of person, a perfectionist who was furious to find herself so crippled at such an early age. She was a starch person – toast, pasta and potatoes made up the bulk of her diet. She did not drink water, only coffee and tea. Like most people with joint problems, her digestion was not robust and she had been constipated for years. Constipation signifies someone who is not digesting their food. In her case the underlying cause of the maldigestion was tension.

Such was the severity of her condition that I could not offer her a choice of treatment. There was only one route and I had to be completely honest with her about what she could expect if she did not accept and stick to the rigid regime I proposed. In the beginning we had many arguments because she found it too difficult. Fortunately, the very stubborn streak in her eventually acted in her best interests and she decided to do all I asked. After three months she could get out of bed and begin tailing back the anti-inflammatory drugs she had been prescribed.

Treatment Plan

The treatment entails changing the acidity inside the joints, principally by eliminating from the diet the worst of the acid-forming foods and using food supplements to make the system more alkaline.

If the problem is severe, eliminate all starches and, depending on how poor the digestion is, other acid foods, such as tomatoes. In less severe cases it is not necessary to be so strict, although bread, potatoes and simple carbohydrates, such as cakes and biscuits, should definitely be excluded.

Start the day by taking 2–3 tablespoons of cider vinegar in warm water; add honey to taste.

Eat mainly vegetables and fruit with small amounts of fish (especially) and chicken. Rice, millet, quinoa and oatbran may also be eaten. But remember never to include both starches and proteins at one meal.

If you are a smoker, try to cut down. Smoking raises the levels of a substance called rheumatoid factor which is associated with the symptoms of joint pain, stiffness and swelling.

Pay particular attention to the volume of each meal (see page 31). It is important that what is eaten is digested properly and does not add to the toxins already in the body.

Take a mild model of digestive enzymes – *Bifidobacterium infantis* (see page 140) – to assist the process of digestion. It is important not to start with a model that is too strong because this may provoke a reaction that makes the joints worse.

Include unsaturated oils in the diet, such as fish oils (cod liver oil or salmon oil, for example), linseed (flax) oil or Udo's oil.

Most people with joint problems are deficient in trace elements due to the acidity in their system hindering absorption. Cal-M (see page 127) makes the system alkaline and assists absorption.

Take Missing Link (see page 138).

Helping Remedies

- Supplements incorporating the vitamins that help combat joint disease (vitamins A, C and D) are available – see entries for Joint Nutrition (page 136), and Lipo-Plex (page 137).
- Take glucosamine sulphate (see page 134) to help joint function and stimulate joint repair, and MSM (see page 138) to reduce pain and inflammation.
- Gentle skin brushing improves the circulation, stimulates the immune system and helps to remove toxins from the body (see page 147).

Helping Therapies

- I would recommend the Pilates method of body conditioning (see page 139) to anybody with joint problems. Cranial or traditional osteopathy treatment also keeps the muscles supple. Water treatment such as floatation therapy is beneficial too, because it relaxes and harmonizes the body.

LOW BLOOD SUGAR

One of the least recognized disorders of modern life – and one of the most common – is hypoglycaemia, or low levels of glucose in the blood. As with most health problems, hypoglycaemia does not just happen to us – we put it on ourselves, through lifestyle and our eating habits. A real danger with low blood sugar is that, if it is not checked, it may eventually lead to diabetes, one of the top ten 'killer' diseases in the West. The low blood sugar brigade – of which I used to be a fully paid up member – invariably suffer with their digestion and health problems hit them earlier than they do most other people. This is not surprising when you consider the way the body is forced to over-run and the strain imposed on it by the constant yo-yoing between high and low levels of glucose in the blood. In the long term such swings put people in serious danger of developing high blood pressure (see page 86) or heart problems.

The body temperature in a hypoglycaemic person is one or two degrees lower than it is in someone with balanced blood sugar, indicating that the immune system is not functioning properly.

The Effect

The simplest cause of low blood sugar is going too long without food. Eating raises the level of glucose in the blood. If we use slow-release foods, such as rice or vegetables, the level rises gradually and does not cross a certain threshold. However, if we take stimulant substances, such as sugary foods, alcohol, nicotine or caffeine, the level of glucose in the blood shoots up. The islets of Langerhans in the pancreas (whose function it is to control sugar and fat metabolism) then respond by producing more insulin to depress the level of glucose. The resulting dip in the blood sugar brings on symptoms ranging from tiredness, hunger, muscular palpitations, depression and shaky hands to anxiety, bad temper, dizziness and headache. The blood pressure drops in tandem with the blood sugar. Unfortunately, because the low blood sugar person tends to have either a 'sweet' or starchy tooth the carbohydrates consumed do not ward off the hunger pangs for long, and so the cycle is repeated in quick succession day in day out.

Are You?

Usually the low blood sugar person is the last to realize he or she has a problem. If you answer 'Yes' to two or more of the following questions, the likelihood is that you are low blood sugar.

Do you often have an irresistible desire to nibble between meals, usually on something sweet or starchy, or a dependence on cigarettes or alcohol to deliver a boost as your mood darkens or energy flags?

Do you find it difficult to stop once you start to nibble, puff or tipple?

Are you ravenous by dinnertime and then tend to over-eat?

Do you tend to be 'flat' in the morning and have to gee yourself up?

Do you eat quickly?

Are you constipated?

Do you tend to skip meals and then feel almost weak or dizzy with hunger?

Do you often feel 'low' and look at yourself hyper-critically?

Do you tend to procrastinate, putting off until the day after tomorrow what could easily be done today?

A Star could be Born

When the glucose level is raised, low blood sugar people are dynamic, amusing, the 'star' in any gathering. When left to their own devices, they tend to be withdrawn, moody, full of self-reproach and, in some cases, self-loathing. When the glucose level starts to swing, they hunt for the biscuit tin, have an alcoholic drink, light a cigarette or take a drug. Non low blood sugar people will get a message to stop, and will be content with one or perhaps two biscuits or drinks. Low blood sugar types get a different message, one encouraging them to over-indulge, especially in those foods or substances that will inevitably make them more toxic.

The low blood sugar type may be characterized as two personalities living in the same body. One side shines like gold and is brilliant with energy and promise; the other is as dull and heavy as lead. Some low blood sugar people are so far out of balance that being alone is unbearable and life only holds any interest when they are at the centre of some self-created drama. This duality creates an inner stress. The tendency to self-denigrate is juxtaposed with feelings of being misunderstood and hard done by. They become frustrated with themselves because they know on the one hand how brilliant they can be and on the other how much of their potential they waste, mainly in futile worry about how they are matching up and what other people are thinking of them.

They are super self-critical, and do not allow for the fact that only machines can be brilliant all the time. They can also tend to be judgmental and short-fused when other people are not prepared – or are unable – to feel their way to a solution and insist instead on using logic. A musical analogy is appropriate here – where the non low blood sugar person will play a piece of music by following a score, the low blood sugar person will improvise. Either approach is valid, and the low blood sugar person has to learn to appreciate that theirs is not the only or best way. There is no shame in having 'off days', when the obvious makes as much sense as a Sanskrit manuscript and the brain seems to be in its equivalent of reverse gear, or in requiring a framework to work or live by, or in being a plodder rather than a meteor. Low blood sugar people are constantly tuned into a memory of past glories when they achieved more and were better. Middle age is a time of increasing irritation with their own perceived – and usually grossly exaggerated – shortcomings. This sense is normally fuelled by the body's diminishing capacity to keep them ahead of the game and the first acknowledgement that all is not well in the health department.

Understanding the Type

Most of the people I treat for low blood sugar came to me in the first instance with some other problem. Low blood sugar is a complication that has to be allowed for in the treatment equation. The patient, too, must be made aware of what it means to have low blood sugar. This is very important, because unless the patient recognizes him- or herself and understands their personality type, treatment may well be impossible.

The low blood sugar person undoubtedly has to work harder at getting well, especially at the outset, and needs ongoing support and encouragement. Some patients I have to telephone every week to see how they are progressing and discuss any problems.When patients start to 'see' themselves, they can counter their negative aspects and cultivate their many good points. I want them to see that they have got a gift, they are like miniature suns, and that life around them can run smoothly and drama-free. And when those negative aspects occasionally get the upper hand, I want them to laugh at themselves before getting back on track with the treatment. One patient, after reaching a better understanding of herself, described very well the typical battle she is waging. She said, 'My cupboards don't talk to me so much any more'.

Low blood sugar people are very sensitive to light, and the lack of warming, cheering sunlight has a depressive effect on them. The months from November to March are especially trying – when this Seasonal Affective Disorder is at its worst – and they have to look after themselves particularly well during this period.

Treatment Plan

The aim of the treatment is to keep the blood sugar even at all times and so reduce the stress imposed by fluctuating glucose levels. The low blood sugar person has to use more guile than most when it comes to tricking the body.

The first trick that has to be learnt is timing. Do not let your blood sugar get low. This means that you have to feed your body every few hours, well before the hunger pangs have reached screaming pitch and driven you to your usual response.

In the beginning, try to have warm food and drinks. These keep the blood sugar raised which in turn keeps the circulation moving and helps to eliminate toxins from the body. When the blood sugar drops, we feel cold. When the digestion improves, the body temperature automatically rises.

Start the day with a cold bath or shower. You will find this purgatory to begin with, but it is a simple, cheap and highly effective way of getting the blood sugar to balance (see page 148). The circulation is the body's merry-go-round. When it is moving well the body's other systems automatically seem to work better.

Have a hot breakfast, perhaps of oatbran porridge with grated apple cooked in it, served with a little honey or cinnamon.

Between meals divert yourself from sweet or starchy foods by offering yourself slow-release foods which take longer to digest than simple carbohydrates and so keep the energy even for longer. Green Energy foods such as chlorella or spirulina will also do this. L-Glutamine (see page 134) taken in a little water is a favourite mid-meal nutrient with some of my patients (although, significantly, not the comfort feeders). Have a bowl of soup (thick vegetable or chicken, for example) mid afternoon as a second lunch or some vegetables left-over from the night before gently heated in stock. Alternatively, you could take some Missing Link (see page 138) in fruit juice. If you are at work, take a thermos flask of soup with you. This will ensure that when you get home in the evening you are not so ravenously hungry that you eat everything in sight. When the blood sugar becomes more balanced, you should be able to survive happily from breakfast to lunch and only need a boost mid-afternoon to carry you through to dinner time.

Do not buy processed foods – these are high in hidden fats and sugars. Unless you can control a tendency to have more than is good for your blood sugar, do not buy cakes, chocolates or sweet biscuits. Reduce, too, the amount of bread you buy.

Low blood sugar people in general do not digest starches well. Avoid complex carbohydrates as much as possible, including potatoes. Rice, millet, quinoa or spelt are the best of these starches, but only if they are eaten in small amounts and chewed well. If they are not, they can make the blood sugar swing as wildly as a bar of chocolate. Avoid, too, sweet fruits such as bananas, dates and raisins.

Try to have your evening meal before 8 o'clock. This will allow you to take some (about a quarter of a tablespoon) Missing Link (see page 138) or a few prunes before bedtime, ensuring that your blood sugar levels are maintained at the right level during the night.

Eat small amounts – remember the volume of your two hands cupped together (see page 31).

If you are constipated, follow the suggestions given on page 76 to make you less so.

Regard the food you have as treats, and think of ways to make the idea of them appeal. Imagine you are at home one afternoon: it is overcast, wet and chilly, the kind of day you hate. In the bad old days your thoughts would probably have roved to the biscuit tin or bread bin. You would have blown yourself out and then felt even more miserable for allowing yourself to get into that state. Today, though, is different. You have put an apple in the oven to bake and when it is ready you will take it out, drizzle some honey over it, sit down and enjoy it. Your comfort will be twofold and derive from the warmth and flavour of the apple and the self-affirmation that eating such wholesome, nutritious food brings. Food does keep body and soul together, and it is important that it should cheer you and make you feel that you are discovering fresh enjoyments.

Helping Remedies

- In cases where the digestion is very poor, digestive enzymes are beneficial (see page 130).
- If your digestion just needs perking up, try drinking ginger and lemon in hot water and the whole lemon and olive oil drink (see page 151 for recipe); both aid digestion. The lemon and olive oil drink will also clean up the liver, raise the body temperature and generally calm the body.

Helping Therapies

- Low blood sugar people respond very well to touch, and any therapy which makes them relax and feel better about their bodies is helpful. Massage, aromatherapy and reflexology are the obvious choices.

Smoke Signal

All smokers have low blood sugar. As we have seen, the effects of smoking are to drain the body on the one hand and stimulate it on the other. Every cigarette smoked takes about 25mg of Vitamin C out of the body. However, if you actually took 25mg of Vitamin C for every cigarette you smoked, you would end up giving yourself diarrhoea and an ulcer. It is sensible to take 2–3mg of slow-release Vitamin C to make up some of this shortfall. Once the blood sugar level balances – through diet – and the body gets more energy and absorbs more nutrients the need to smoke will lessen

ME

We all know what it feels like to be hung over. ME sufferers feel that way every day. I regard ME as a form of viral or microbial disorder, like herpes and hepatitis, and akin to self-poisoning. A virus may be described as microorganisms living in your space which will blossom when the conditions are right.

All the ME sufferers I have treated have had low blood sugar (see page 102), and the majority of them have taken too many courses of antibiotics. Our response to antibiotics depends largely on how well we are, and our degree of sensitivity to them. It is not known for sure what effect antibiotics have on the immune system or why some people are more sensitive to them. My hunch is that in someone who is already fermenting badly because of poor digestion, antibiotics encourage a build-up of undigested food. The toxicity arising from this erodes the gut wall, allowing large molecules of incompletely digested matter to enter the bloodstream. This is the starting point of the allergies that seem to characterize ME and other auto-immune diseases. The polluting spores which inhabit the sufferer's immune system burst into full bloom when the person becomes run down or over-tired. The problem is compounded by the taking of subsequent courses of antibiotics to kill the virus. The more antibiotics we take, the worse the fermentation in the gut and the 'leakier' or more prone to recurring infections or viruses we become.

ME and its viral partners enmesh the sufferer in a continually evolving maze of illness from which it is very difficult to escape. The body is under constant attack, but because its immune system has been so severely degraded, it is incapable of fighting back with sufficient vigour to see off the threat once and for all. Viruses represent the constant tread of the degeneration process; the hepatitis virus, for example, is increasingly being seen as a precursor to certain kinds of cancer.

Profile

Given the debilitating nature of ME it is not surprising that sufferers have little energy or enthusiasm. Everything is difficult, including getting better. This is particularly problematical and patients can find themselves in a catch-22 situation. Changing the flora has to be done very, very slowly if the bacteria killed off in the process of clearing the body are not to cause a healing crisis or worse. A patient of mine who was frustrated by the rate of progress went for colonic irrigation and felt decidedly worse afterwards as a result of the toxic matter stirred up by the treatment. Colonic cleansing can be extremely beneficial but if it is done too vigorously it can expose the body to a healing crisis, as occurred in this case.

People who suffer from ME or any other sort of viral disorder have to accept that they are living in a low-energy body. Depression is never far away because of the limits imposed on them. Everyday pleasures, such as taking a walk or going out to a concert or the cinema, are denied to many sufferers, who understandably resent their predicament. Finding ways to overcome the lack of motivation or desire which their situation encourages is an important strand of treatment. Sufferers must try to broaden the feasible options within what at times probably seems like a shrinking personal world – and be kind to themselves.

What drains you? If someone is nagging you or knocking your confidence, make a decision to see less of that person. Choose friends who will not deplete your energy further, but will rather boost your self-esteem and make you feel positive about yourself.

What cheers you up and makes you laugh? Do you like singing or movement? Perhaps you like to watch or read comedy. Try to introduce new interests that will relax you and put you in an optimistic frame of mind.

Treatment Plan

The aim in treating ME and similar viral conditions is to rebuild the immune system and the protective membrane or buffer between the gut and the lymphatic. A strict diet is necessary, although unlikely to yield a discernible improvement for weeks, possibly months. For the ME sufferer, just thinking about food, let alone preparing a meal, is likely to be difficult, so to begin with confine yourself to eating very simple, easy to digest foods, such as lightly cooked vegetables in stock, chicken or gluten-free quinoa-pasta or rice with vegetables.

Everything you eat must be aimed at achieving the goal of making the digestive system alkaline. This will not be easy because ME sufferers tend to like starch and sugar; see the list of alkali-forming foods given on page 62 for alternatives to these.

Assess how you are digesting your food. Pay particular attention to the volume you eat at each meal and chewing each mouthful thoroughly.

Foods containing sugar should be eliminated. Sugar stops the immune system functioning.

Get the acidity in the mouth right, using the whole lemon and olive oil drink (see page 151 for recipe). Buy pH strips to check your progress (see page 147).

Ensure that your foods and drinks are warm to raise the body temperature and further aid digestion.

Helping Remedies

- Sage and thyme strengthen the immune system. They can be taken as herbal teas. The herb echinacea and the tonic Shou Wu Chih are also helpful in increasing the body's immunity, as is Essiac tea (see pages 130, 131 and 142).
- Take a cold bath or shower each day to increase the circulation and thus the immune system (see page 148).

Helping Therapies

- Chelation or oxygen treatment is especially appropriate for people with viral disorders. It is not widely available but worthwhile seeking out (see page 128).
- Slow cleaning of the colon is always helpful and many patients find colonic irrigation beneficial. Some practitioners, however, are reluctant to treat people in whom the overgrowth is very severe because the treatment has to proceed so slowly that results are hard to judge and few people have the patience to receive weeks of what may seem to them like no treament at all.

MIGRAINE

A migraine is more than a blinding headache, as sufferers will confirm. The body gives off warning signals when an attack is imminent, the most common being bright lights appearing before the sufferer's eyes and a feeling of sickness. A migraine attack can leave some people unable to function – sight, speech and motor skills may all be seriously affected. It is as though the body is short-circuiting. To my mind, this is exactly what is happening.

Profile

In most migraine sufferers I have treated the digestion has been out of sorts for some time. They are either constipated or have deteriorated a stage further into diarrhoea and irritable bowel-type symptoms (see page 96). Migraine is in the same area of the health ball park as high blood pressure and high cholesterol and it is not unusual for sufferers to develop one or both of these other conditions.

Migraine sufferers tend to work too hard, too long, usually in stressful jobs. A great deal of this stress may arise from the fact that they feel constantly on display, under scrutiny or open to criticism. They live on their adrenaline, which tricks the body into staying in fifth gear, enabling them to keep surging ahead. Typically, when they start to come down through the gears and the pressure they put on themselves is eased, the body judders and rebels, rewarding them with a migraine. This usually happens on the third day when their energy has dropped to zero as the adrenaline is withdrawn. If you are a migraine sufferer, recall how many times you have experienced an attack at the tail end of a weekend or on a Monday morning.

Statistically more women than men get migraines. In some of my women patients the precipitating factor would appear to be a dip in the level of the hormone progesterone which lowers the blood sugar. In this pattern the migraine usually occurs one or two days before a period. If this is your experience with migraine, try taking wild yam one to two weeks before your period is due to lift the progesterone level. If you are in any doubt about how to proceed, consult a therapist.

In children, migraine is usually a symptom of hyperactivity; I define a hyperactive child as one who does not eat vegetables, and has a liking for sharp, sugary and artificial foods.

I have yet to treat an elderly person for migraines. I put this down to the fact that by this stage in life we are no longer striving and so the emotional strains and stresses which precipitate this condition have fallen away. In my experience, the most important factor in migraine is the individual's sensitivity to stress and his or her ability to cope with it.

Treatment Plan

Follow the Basic Programme (see page 55) with these modifications for three weeks or until the migraines cease and you feel better. The treatment is intended to make you more aware of how your body is feeling, so that in future you will be able to recognize the signs – for example, putting on weight or feeling as though life is running away from you – and take avoiding action. You will soon develop a sixth sense that tells you when they are in danger from your old habits. When you get these signs, revert to the diet and start to clear up the body again.

In many migraine sufferers constipation has been caused by eating too much, too quickly while tense. Eating habits, therefore, must be addressed and special care taken to sit down to eat, chew each mouthful well, and relax during and after eating.

For breakfast, grate one green apple the night before in order to allow the fruit to brown. Avoid other fruit, apart from papaya and pineapple (both of these are good for the digestion), which would ferment too much at this stage. If constipated, top the apple with one tablespoon of soaked linseed. Drink a cup of ginger or green tea – avoid coffee and ordinary tea.

For lunch and dinner, eat protein and vegetables; for example, grilled or poached fish and grilled or casseroled chicken with steamed vegetables. At the end of the treatment, starches can be reintroduced, but at this juncture it is advisable to avoid these acid-forming foods.

Take ginger and lemon tea, vegetable stock, light vegetable soup, Missing Link (see page 138) in fruit juice or Green Energy (see page 135) foods mid-afternoon in order to maintain your energy levels.

Throughout the day, but preferably between meals, drink 3 litres (5 pints) of water.

In the evening take Cal-M (see page 127).

Drink milk thistle tea (see page 137).

Limit the drinking of traditional tea and especially coffee to one cup of each per day.

Danger Foods

Try to permanently eliminate the following from your diet – cow's milk, cheese, foods containing gluten, chocolate, coffee, Diet Coke and similar soft drinks.

Helping Remedies

- If you find it particularly difficult to unwind and are thus prone to blocking your digestion through tension, use enzymes to assist the process of digestion. Chamomile tincture will also help in this respect.
- The herbal tincture feverfew is helpful as a preventative.
- Dr Reckeweg's complex homeopathic remedy for migraine, R 16.

Helping Therapies

- Cranial osteopathy. In some sufferers the cause of migraines is mechanical, perhaps due to pressure on the skull during birth or a later misalignment of the spine. If you suspect such an injury, it may be worthwhile having yourself checked over by a qualified therapist. Even if neither of these is the case, cranial osteopathy is excellent for balancing the body; after such treatment you should feel your energy reviving.
- Investigate therapies that will help you to relax, such as reflexology, body harmony in salt water, aromatherapy, or anything else that appeals.
- The essential oils lavender, grapefruit and marjoram rubbed into the body, especially the temples, can have a beneficial effect.

PANIC ATTACKS

Panic attacks are caused by the adrenaline overshooting as a result of the body being subjected to years of stress and being pushed too hard. The person will probably have received warning signs in the form of moodiness or excessive anxiety. Most people who experience panic attacks are of the low blood sugar type (see page 102) who have not taken steps to ensure that the glucose in the blood is kept even. If the signs are not heeded, suddenly he or she will find themselves no longer in control, unable to breathe, their heart beating against their chest alarmingly, and generally unable to cope. A panic attack can also be brought on by an excess of alcohol, caffeine or drugs.

Profile

Many people who experience panic attacks are their own worst enemy, tending to live on their nerves and not knowing how to be laid back. They inhabit a body that is exhausted and in desperate need of rest, and a mind that needs to be at peace with itself. Unfortunately, many of them seem incapable of learning how to use all their 'gears', and of varying the pace and intensity of life.

Panic attacks can occur in people who by most yardsticks would be regarded as living in a stress-free zone. One of my patients did not have to work for a living, and she was financially very comfortable, but she was a very 'busy' individual. Her panic attacks came on after her dog died, when at a stroke she lost her excuse for busyness and a meaningful routine. Instead of taking him to the park every morning, she became the bane of the assistants in Harrods, running in and out of the shop, making purchases, returning them, then buying something else, and so on. This became a full-time job: she did not have time for lunch or to relax. If she sat down, she could not concentrate; or if she tried to cook a meal she would become totally confused.

The anxiety which fuels panic attacks can be generated by seemingly trivial matters, such as fear of saying 'No' to another person or not wanting to do something. In very bad cases a fleeting thought about the underlying fear or worry can trigger an attack and, as a consequence, can prevent the person dealing with that underlying problem, thus compounding it. If an attack is used as an excuse not to do something the situation will progressively worsen.

This layering effect was noticeable in a woman who came to see me about her panic attacks. Unbeknown to me she was using alcohol to calm herself down and was in danger of becoming an alcoholic. She had reached the stage where she could not face doing anything – from shopping for groceries to attending a dinner party – without first having a drink. The alcohol made her panic attacks worse in the long run; rather than calming her down they had the effect of initially cranking her up and later dropping her into a deep pit of depression.

We started the treatment with the aim of getting her digestion right. Most people who suffer panic attacks have diarrhoea and I made it a priority to remedy this. The view that panic attacks are all in the mind is not uncommon, but to my way of thinking the top brain is only partly to blame. The role of the lower brain in the gut should not be ignored. We worked on her diet for 6 to 8 weeks. At the end of this period she was experiencing fewer panic attacks. About four months later she realized that she was no longer as dependent on alcohol to see her through difficult situations. It took a further year for her to reach the stage where she is now, not dependent on it at all.

Treatment Plan

In addition to following the Basic Programme (see page 55) it is also important to confront the problem underlying the attacks and find ways of solving that. This may entail looking at what is important in your life and reassessing your situation and your relationships. If you find yourself becoming agitated over irrelevancies, such as dirt on the carpet, dust on the furniture or someone walking or driving slowly in front of you, stop and think. Your body does not need unnecessary pressure of this sort to build up and feed on itself.

Because panic attacks leave the body feeling very flat, a priority is to keep the energy even at all times. Eat little and often and break the common pattern of eating either too much or nothing at all. Eating too much at one go can bring on a panic attack as well as overload the system.

Have warm rather than cold food to encourage your system to relax and also to aid digestion.

Eliminate foods that have a fast insulin response, such as sugar, coffee, chocolate and bread.

Helping Remedies

- There are various homeopathic remedies, such as hypericum and valerian, to calm the nerves; the relaxant kava-kava (see page 136) is also helpful. However, the most complete benefit is to be had from Cal-M (see page 127). If this is sipped throughout the day, it will nourish and calm the system.

- If insomnia is a problem, see that treatment (page 95).

Helping Therapies

- Most people who suffer with panic attacks do not breathe properly. They are what I call 'hoverers' and breathe shallowly. The most beneficial therapy, therefore, is deep breathing allied to meditation. Learning how to breathe properly can be problematic, because rarely are you sure that you are doing it correctly. There is a machine that teaches you how to breathe properly and gives feedback so you can monitor your progress (see page 126).

PMS

Most women are not in such good shape that they do not experience some PMS symptoms. Some women suffer badly, experiencing headaches as well as pains elsewhere in the body and moodiness. In other women it may be only their partners or children who recognize the signs of tetchiness and instant exasperation.

Most PMS sufferers have low blood sugar (see page 102), and they tend to eat too much. When the blood sugar drops, fewer digestive enzymes are made and as a consequence the digestion is less efficient than usual; usual efficiency in low blood sugar women corresponds to well below par in non low blood sugar women. Incorrect fermentation causes the characteristic bloated stomach that many sufferers experience about a week before the start of their period. A badly acidic system will also cause the sufferer to have weak nails and hair, and impair absorption. Many PMS sufferers are low in prostaglandins, which are vital for regulating hormonal activity, and as a consequence too much of the hormone prolactin is produced.

Treatment Plan

PMS cannot occur if the fermentation in the colon is right and the blood sugar is kept even. This can be achieved by making the system more alkaline and nourishing it with slow-release foods; many women with

PMS tend to crave sugar or chocolate, foods that exacerbate the underlying problem. The basics of sensible eating must be understood and followed if PMS is to become a memory.

Follow the diet given in the treatment plan under Low Blood Sugar (see page 102).

Choose foods that are alkali-forming (see page 62) – the more quickly the system becomes alkaline the less of a problem PMS will be. Alkalinity is also assisted by a high intake of the essential fatty acids found in flax oil and Udo's oil (see page 144).

Gamma-linolenic acid, in the form of evening primrose oil, will help to smooth out the hormonal swings and calm production of prolactin.

Helping Remedies

- The herbal tonic Shou Wu Chih is helpful.

Helping Therapies

- Most PMS sufferers respond well to hands-on, energy-giving treatments, such as aromatherapy massage, acupuncture and reflexology.

SKIN DISORDERS

The skin is a mirror of the gut. Dry, blotchy, flaky or spotty skin are overflows from a badly fermenting, toxic digestive system.

A skin disorder signifies that the whole 'pond' is dirty. Antibiotics can keep the problem under control, but once they are withdrawn the condition will return, often with a vengeance. By increasing the toxicity in the body, antibiotics make the situation worse and patients who have been on them for a long time are without doubt the most difficult to treat.

In my experience most people who suffer with bad skin have low blood sugar. They love starch foods, such as potatoes, bread and chocolate, and eat too much of them. This excess builds up in the system as toxins. Of course, if they had small helpings and chewed the food to perfection, the starches would be pre-digested in the mouth and this build up would not occur.

The condition of the skin will only begin to improve when the fermentation and the functioning of the gut are corrected by bringing the microflora back into balance and facilitating the absorption of trace elements and vitamins. If the skin is weeping, extra care has to be taken to eliminate all acid-forming foods from the diet – not one teaspoonful of sugar should find its way into the sufferer's system. The reason for such strictness is explained by the following story.

Profile

A 25-year-old man came to me with puffy skin covered in weeping sores. He had a history of poor skin but it was only after he had been in a very stressful job for a while that it developed into such an obvious problem. He had been living alone on a diet high in beer and carbohydrates. When he came to see me he had been forced to give up his job and had returned home to his parents. He had reached the stage with his diet where even relatively small amounts of starch, such as in root vegetables or potatoes, was making the problem worse. It seemed to me that over-consumption of starch had made him allergic to it.

I put him on the most boring diet imaginable: chicken soup, grated apple and lightly cooked green vegetables. In addition, he had a high intake of linseed oil, and underwent gentle colonic irrigation. He had a very sweet tooth, and the one element of cheer I allowed him in his bleak dietary routine was a cup of tea with sweetener; even honey blew him up. Slowly he began to get better. One day he phoned me in a state of panic, and said, 'Gudrun, I can feel my skin burning'. I asked him what he had been doing. He insisted that he had not deviated from the programme he had been following for the past three months. It turned out that his mother had run out of the sweetener and, not thinking it could possibly harm him, had added one small teaspoonful of cane sugar to his tea.

Treatment Plan

Initially the pattern of treatment will be determined by the nature of each sufferer's weak digestion. Sufferers would be wise to look at how they digest their food. For example, tense individuals will need to find ways of not blocking their digestion – remember the link between the two brains. Emotional upsets or stress cause the system to release adrenaline and divert it from the job of digesting the food being put into it. The skin will only improve and get a better texture when this problem has been resolved.

Most people with skin problems are either constipated or have irritable bowel syndrome. Follow the relevant programme (see pages 75 and

96) for at least one week before beginning the treatment given below.

All other skin sufferers should follow the Basic Programme (page 55) for 2 to 3 weeks. In addition, eliminate foods that are acid-forming or ferment badly, such as chocolate, cheese, cane sugar (substitute honey) and bread.

To help the on-going process of detoxification, get oxygen into the system to kill off the bad bacteria by eating grated apple that has been allowed to go black. This is an effective anti-fungal method which changes the fermentation in the gut. Apple prepared in this way can be taken two or three times each day. However, monitor its effect – the amount and frequency will vary from person to person, and the last thing you want to provoke is a reaction.

The microorganisms which are supposed to break down our food and help us absorb nutrients are absent in people with severe skin disorders. Patients have to slowly build an army of good bacterial flora. After one week of following the treatment measures, introduce a mild model (suitable for children) of Acidophilus (see page 139), then change to a stronger model. It is very important to test and monitor this process. If you experience a reaction, such as headaches, giddiness, itchiness or a skin eruption, perhaps even panic attacks, you will know the model is too strong and that you need to build more slowly.

Take the whole lemon and olive oil drink (see page 151 for recipe).

Take a balance of omega-3 and omega-6 unsaturated oils, such as Udo's oil (see page 144).

Helping Remedies

- For psoriasis, try Dr Reckeweg's R 65 homeopathic complex.
- If the skin is dry and itchy, try aloe vera gel or cream, or adding a quarter of a cup of cider vinegar to your bath.
- Try gentle skin brushing (see page 147) – although not directly on the affected area or areas. This will help the body rid itself of toxins (and thus the problem) by stimulating the circulation.

Helping Therapies

- Bath in salts (Dead Sea salts are the strongest), which will pull the toxins through the skin. Afterwards apply a soothing yet cleansing vegetable-based cream or oil, such as aloe vera; Udo's oil can be used effectively for this purpose, too.

ULCER

Gastric ulcers were until recently thought to be caused by an excess of stomach acid secreted in response to stress or too much fatty food. A bacterium that inflames the stomach lining, *Helicobacter pylori*, is now known to be the real culprit in many cases, and is also thought by some specialists to induce stomach cancer. This occurs as a result of malfunction in the digestive system.

An ulcer can form in any part of the body, from the mouth to the small intestine, bladder or kidney. I regard an ulcer as a fungal blossoming, signifying a weakness at the point it appears in the gel lining the digestive tract. A simple mouth ulcer, for example, would not arise if the saliva was sufficiently alkaline. Eating large quantities of sugar or chocolate will encourage the growth of an ulcer by altering the delicate acid/alkaline balance. If this imbalance occurs further down in the system, for example in the stomach, incorrect fermentation may create conditions favourable to a serious fungal blossoming in, say, the duodenum.

Profile

Most people who develop ulcers tend to eat too much and thus create a pool of undigested food in the system. This tendency coupled with a refusal to recognize that their digestion is their weak point means that they are perpetually compounding the problem. The situation is exacerbated when they are put under pressure by life's worries, for invariably they react by eating even more, adding to the already considerable stress on their digestive system.

Many patients find it difficult to accept that the whole system has to be calmed down in order for the ulcer to heal properly, and that they cannot expect to return to bad eating habits even when the ulcer is clinically regarded as 'cured'. One patient of mine had received treatment for a duodenal ulcer and then been told that nothing could be done about her stomach distending and causing great discomfort. Her diet seemed to consist of beans, lentils and bread, so to my way of thinking the cause of her problem was straightforward enough. She agreed to reduce the size of her meals, to chew her food thoroughly, to eat easily-digestible foods, and to aid the digestive system with enzymes. However, when she realized that bread fell into the category of difficult-to-digest and would have to be given up, she refused the treament. She reasoned that bread had been eaten for thousands of years, it was a staple food and that by definition it was good for us.

It took several arguments to convince her that bread had only to be banished until the ulcer was better. Eventually, she agreed to do as I advised for one week, and for the duration of that week she ate nothing but small, frequent meals of lightly cooked green vegetables, chewed well. At the end of the week the wind was greatly reduced and she felt she had taken a small step forward. After three months she went to her GP to tell him how much better she was. Three months on she came back to me complaining that the treatment had failed because the bloating and discomfort had returned. When I asked about her diet she admitted that she had reverted to her old ways of eating one large meal a day. We corrected the acid/alkaline balance and built up the good gut flora once more, and I am reasonably confident that she has understood what she has to do in order to keep herself well.

In this the last treatment, it is appropriate to underline a theme running through this book. If, as most of the treatments indicate, the system has been fermenting badly for many years, we cannot expect to revert to unwise eating habits and remain well. We must look after ourselves as well in good health as we do in bad.

Treatment Plan

At whatever point in the system an ulcer appears, the priority is to alter the alakaline/acid balance to enable it to heal and to prevent the development of microorganisms in the digestive system. Any ulcer, specially in the digestive system, requires a return to babyhood for several weeks. Once an ulcer has been diagnosed most sufferers are prescribed drugs that work on the brain to halt the release of acid in the stomach. The wise person will regard such drugs as short-term aids to enable the ulcer to heal. This will only happen, however, if during this period only bland or pre-digested food that does not stimulate the acidity is eaten, and the sufferer helps the process by chewing all food to perfection. Continuance of the bad habits that produced the ulcer in the first place will make the situation worse and may possibly lead to a more serious problem.

Return to the basics, looking at the volume of each meal and how you can create the conditions for good digestion – see page 27 if you need to refresh your memory. Remember that acid-forming foods can be transformed by thorough chewing. Thorough chewing will also ensure that there are no particles of undigested matter to irritate the ulcer.

Eliminate the worst of the acid-forming foods, such as products containing gluten (especially wheat), cheese and tomatoes. (See the lists of acid-forming and alkali-forming foods on page 62.)

Eat very little protein, restricting yourself to foods that are easy to digest, such as chicken soup, chicken stock, fish. In addition, eat steamed, baked or stir-fried vegetables. Papaya and stewed apple are the two fruits most helpful to an ulcer.

All vegetables should be cooked slightly. Raw food will tend to scuff the ulcer and hinder the healing process.

Eliminate coffee, which tends to strip the gel lining the system. Alcoholic drinks, too, are irritants and should be avoided.

Eliminate spicy foods and foods that are high in saturated fats.

L-Glutamine (see page 134) sipped in water between meals will help to heal the lining. Start with a quarter of a teaspoon per dose and gradually progress to three teaspoons. Monitor its effect; if you find it constipating, reduce the dose.

Aloe vera is helpful, but must be well diluted so it does not aggravate the ulcer.

After one or two weeks of following the treatment, introduce a mild (suitable for children) model of milk-free Acidophilus (see page 139) in powder form on food to help the bacterial flora.

Helping Remedies

- Any herbal tea that calms the stomach, such as peppermint, marshmallow and slippery elm, or chamomile will be beneficial.
- If you have a very tense stomach, relax for as long as possible after meals to aid digestion. A hot water bottle placed against the back can have a very relaxing and calming effect on the system.

Helping Therapies

- Any calming therapy that reduces stress is beneficial, such as reflexology, aromatherapy or massage.

NO-FRILLS OPTION

Whatever your state of health, if by any chance you reach the conclusion that, 'No, this is too difficult. I can't do it', consider the following series of simple, low-cost measures.

Take one tablespoon of cider vinegar in warm water and honey in the morning to alkalize the system. Alternatively, take BioCarbonate, a mixture of carbonates (sodium and potassium) which allow the digestive enzymes to perform their function at the correct pH (acid/alakaline) balance.

For breakfast, have cooked oatbran with grated apple.

Cook the tops of green vegetables to a pulp and sip the liquer extracted from them mid- morning and afternoon. This will help your intake of trace elements. In spring, make a vegetable stock from the first growth of nettles; at this time of year these are tender and taste like spinach.

Do not eat starch and protein at the same meal.

Check the volume you eat at each meal – remember the two cupped hands principle (see page 31).

Take Cal-M (see page 127) to feed the liver.

Aid the fermentation in the gut by taking low-strength milk-free Acidophilus (*Bifidobacterium infantis*) or a small amount of Sauerkraut juice before meals.

Take the whole lemon and olive oil drink (see page 151 for recipe) each day to maintain the immune system.

Chapter Five

FOODS, SUPPLEMENTS AND REMEDIES

Acidophilus – see Probiotics

Algae

Algae are non-flowering water plants which are rich sources of chlorophyll, the substance that gives plants their green colour and enables them to use the energy of the sun to create their food. They contain a little of almost all the vitamins, trace elements and minerals we need, and are especially rich in iron. Algae are, in fact, the most nutrient-dense foods on earth. Collectively they are responsible for 90 per cent of the earth's oxygen production and 80 per cent of its food supply. There are estimated to be about 50,000 species of algae. The oldest forms of algae are the freshwater groups, such as blue-green algaes. Seaweed and plankton are examples of seawater algaes.

Algae is at the bottom of the food chain, and is thus thought to be the purest source of nutrients available to us. The concentration of toxins and pollutants increases with each additional link in the food chain. Man is at the top of this chain and his food contains all the accumulated toxins from the agents that have gone into making the chain. Algae is the highest vegetable source of B12 (vital for vegetarians), the richest known source of chlorophyll (a cell regenerator and blood purifier), it contains both proteins and carbohydrates in easily assimiliable forms, it contains active enzymes necessary for its complete absorption by the body, it is a source of nucleic and fatty acids, and it is alkalizing.

Spirulina and chlorella are forms of algae, as are Japanese dried sea vegetables such as nori and wakame. Quality can vary between algae products, so ensure that the one you choose is of high-quality and organic. Eat small amounts of algae to begin with – treat it as you would a new remedy, one that may cause a healing crisis if you push on too enthusiastically.

Aloe vera

Aloe vera has been used for over 2,000 years to soothe and heal bites, stings, burns and skin conditions such a eczema and psoriasis. More recently it has been shown to provide much wider benefits. Aloe contains polysaccharides and prostaglandins. The former are highly beneficial to the digestive system, enhancing digestion and the absorption of food, and reducing bacterial pollution in the gut. Prostaglandins are found in many body tissues where they perform multiple functions, from reducing inflammation to balancing the hormone system and blood sugar levels. Aloe has also been found to be beneficial in the treatment of viruses and auto-immune disorders.

Angelica

Angelica is used in the treatment of indigestion and wind, as well as colds, coughs, pleurisy, rheumatism and diseases of the urinary organs. It is not suitable for those with a tendency towards diabetes, because it causes an increase of sugar in the urine.

Aniseed (Anise)

The oil made from the seeds of this eastern Mediterranean plant is good for wind, slight constipation, coughs and, in children, catarrh. The plant's principal active constituent, anethol, stimulates all glands. It is rather nice to chew aniseed seeds after a meal to clear the palate.

Apple

Apple is a cleanser and balancer, thanks to its contents of pectin, Vitamin C and malic and tartaric acids. Pectin binds to toxins in the body and carries them out of the system. The malic and tartaric acids neutralize the by-products of indigestion and reduce the effects of rich or fatty foods. Any digestive problems or infections are helped by eating apple.

Prepare apple for breakfast the night before, to allow it to go brown and oxidate. The darker the flesh of the apple becomes the more powerful the anti-fungal properties it has gathered. Eating an oxidated apple is a cheap and effective way of taking oxygen into the body and killing off fungi or toxins in the gut.

Never peel an apple, otherwise the beneficial effect of the pectin will be lost, so make sure your apple is organic – and green. Red apples do not contain the same kind of liver-stimulating pectin and therefore do not have the same strong effect. A reaction to the pectin in apple indicates an irritated gall bladder.

Barley

This cereal has been in cultivation longer than any other: barley bread was a staple in the Middle Ages until it was superceded by bread made with oats and then wheat. Barley contains high levels of potassium, calcium and many of the B-complex vitamins. Barley water (not to be confused with the popular drink of the same name) is helpful in cystitis, constipation, in inflammatory digestive conditions, and for convalescents or those suffering fatigue or stress. A low-sugar drink called barley cup which has a similar effect is available from health-food stores.

Beta-carotene

Beta-carotene is a branch of the Vitamin A family and is partially converted by the intestinal mucous membrane to this vitamin. An important anti-oxidant, it is thought to be responsible for the protective effect against cancer found in fruit and vegetables. Carrots, spinach and broccoli are rich in beta-carotene. Even large amounts of beta-carotene can not result in Vitamin A poisoning, because the body breaks down only the amount it requires.

Bifidobacterium – see Probiotics

Boswellia

Also known as Indian frankincense, Boswellia comes from the Ayurvedic tradition of medicine. It is excellent for joint conditions, especially arthritis, and works by inhibiting the synthesis of substances called leukotrines which trigger inflammation. Boswellia is also effective in lowering cholesterol and protecting the liver.

Breathing Machine

Breathing properly does not come naturally. Most people breathe shallowly and are less healthy as a consequence because by reducing the amount of oxygen we take into the body we enable harmful bacteria to flourish. Correct breathing technique has to be taught, which is why I recommend a device – called the Powerbreathe – developed by the University of Birmingham. This hand-held device improves breathing capacity by exercising and strengthening the chest muscles. Several of my patients have improved their lung function considerably by using it for just a few minutes each day.

Cal-M

I suggest Cal-M for a wide range of health problems because of its stabilizing effect on the acid/alkaline balance and the all-round benefits it confers. It is an instant drink powder containing calcium gluconate, magnesium carbonate and organic apple cider vinegar. The mild acidity of the cider vinegar converts the calcium and magnesium into soluble acetate forms, ensuring their effective absorption by the digestive system. Potassium, phosphorous and the trace elements zinc and iron are also provided by the cider vinegar.

In Cal-M magnesium and calcium work in tandem, balancing each other and working with other nutrients in the body to combat free radicals (see page 25). As well as being essential to the absorption of calcium, magnesium is now recognized as a key nutrient in fighting stress. Calcium promotes bone formation, regulates the heart and its functions, and the activity of the muscles and the nervous system. The benefits of taking Cal-M are especially appropriate to older women in whom, without supplementation, calcium is excreted during the night, leading to a loss of bone density.

In cases where the stomach is weak an even gentler option than Cal-M is Biocare's Citrase preparation. In this combination of calcium and magnesium the two minerals are bonded to citric acid to form citrates which provide high levels of absorption. Citrase also provides plant-derived enzymes to assist digestion and boron proteinate to support the skeletal structure.

Candistatin

Prepared by Bio-Care, this combination of the anti-fungal South American plant Pau D'Arco, freeze dried garlic, the alkaloid berberine (which helps normalize the natural bacterial content of the gut, and supports and activates the immune system) and silymarin, detoxifies the bowel. Its use is appropriate in cases of slight constipation where the build-up of toxins in the system is not too great.

Chamomile (Matricaria chamomilla)

German or wild chamomile has a wide range of medicinal uses. The first part of its Latin name (*Matricaria* comes from matrix, meaning womb) indicates one of the plant's principal uses since ancient times. Chamomile tea is generally soothing to the digestive system and the stomach.

Charcoal

Charcoal powder, granules or tablets are prepared from vegetable matter such as peat, cellulose residues and coconut shells. The medicinal value of charcoal lies in its ability to absorb intestinal gases and, in cases of poisoning, drugs such as aspirin, paracetemol, barbiturates and morphine.

Cheese

The strength of cheese as a food is often overlooked, and so it is not surprising that it gives many people indigestion. If we were presented with meat composed of 60 per cent fat, we would not eat it, yet the high fat content of cheese deters few people. Cow protein is not easily broken down by humans, and leads to blocking of the lymphatic system. Cheese made with goat's and ewe's milk is not as bad in this respect, but there is no escaping the fact that it is animal fat too. Cheese is also difficult to chew thoroughly and so tends to land in the gut in big lumps. If you want to eat it, choose a low-fat variety, preferably made from goat's or ewe's milk, make sure you chew it well and serve it with vegetables, not bread.

Chelation

Chelation comes from the Greek word 'chele' and literally means 'to grab hold of'. In this treatment a chelating agent, such as the trace element potassium, is put into the body intravenously to draw out toxic substances, such as heavy metals and mineral deposits. The treatment helps to cleanse the arteries and veins as well as to detoxify the liver and kidneys. It is particularly appropriate for circulatory disorders, such as high cholesterol. The treatment is only available from chelation therapy clinics and can not be self-administered.

Chlorella – see Algae

Chromium

This essential trace mineral plays an important role in our immune system and also in making insulin work more effectively in regulating blood sugar. Research has revealed a connection between chromium deficiency and the risk of coronary vascular disorders. The official recommended daily allowance for chromium set by the World Health Organization is 50–200 micrograms. The average Northern European diet contains between 30 to 40 micrograms. Research shows that only in India is intake of chromium adequate (c. 140 micrograms).

Meat, shellfish (especially mussels), wholemeal and brewer's yeast are relatively high in chromium. However, even with a good diet it is difficult to get near the 125 micrograms daily intake recommended by the WHO. The chromium content in food is affected by how that food is prepared. Losses are caused by heating and industrial processing, and little or no chromium is to be found in grilled, frozen or ready prepared foods.

Chromium supplements are available. Choose organic chromium, also called chromium yeast, in preference to inorganic chromium. The body will absorb less than one per cent of the amount of the latter taken. Dietary fibre increases the body's ability to absorb and utilize chromium.

Cider Vinegar

Cider vinegar is made from the juice of fermented apples and contains small amounts of the minerals potassium and calcium. It is an all-round health supplement and system-balancer: it relieves the symptoms of arthritis, stimulates the liver to produce more bile, thus aiding digestion, inhibits intestinal infections and helps to regulate metabolism.

If you have an acid or sensitive system, take cider vinegar in its gentler, dried form (powder or capsules) – see Cal-M on page 127. Taken in its liquid form, it may make some sensitive stomachs burn slightly.

Crateagus (Hawthorn)

Crataegus tincture is useful in the treatment of heart conditions and those involving the circulation. It gently dilates the coronory vessels, thus increasing the supply of blood to the heart and enhancing the utilization of oxygen in the body.

Croisia – see Milk Thistle

Dill

The word dill is said to come from the old Norse word 'dilla', meaning 'to lull'. The fruit and oil of the plant possess stimulant, aromatic, anti-flatulence and digestion-promoting properties.

Echinacea purpurea (Purple cone flower)

This has been used for hundreds of years as a blood purifier and cleanser. Echinacea works by stimulating the body's white blood cells, the cells of the immune system which help us fight infection. It is effective against viruses, bacteria and fungi.

Elderberry Extract

This extract, taken from the black Elder tree (*Sambuca nigra*), has been found to be highly effective against all types of flu virus. The active extract of elderberry binds to the tiny spikes with which viruses attack the body cells and prevent them from taking hold. Elderberry is also effective against the herpes, Epstein-Barr and HIV viruses.

Elderflower

Taken as an infusion this plant is an excellent blood purifier. It is helpful in colds, flu and for sore throats and has a gently laxative effect. The flowers of the plant can be used externally for piles, boils and skin problems.

Enzymes

Digestive enzymes can be taken before each meal to aid the complete breakdown of food and thus ensure maximum absorption of nutrients. They are particularly appropriate if the body's own production of enzymes is low, because of illness or increasing age, for example; the natural production of digestive enzymes declines progressively from middle age. Manufactured enzymes were at one time only available from pancreatin, an animal product. Now carbohydrate-, fat- and protein-ingesting enzymes are available in the same capsule.

As with Acidophilus, always start with the mildest enzyme. I use a broad spectrum complex of plant origin called Enzyme Aid which helps with the efficient digestion of fats, proteins and carbohydrates. Slightly stronger are Udo's Digestive Enzymes and, if bloating and constipation are present, Biocare's combination Hcl (hydrochloric acid) and Pepsin. If constipation is slight, try a blend of herbs and enzymes, such as Candistatin, which aids the digestion while also helping gentle natural elimination of the bowels.

Essential Fatty Acids (EFAs)

These are called essential because we can not survive without them. EFAs pick up base toxins and balance the cholesterol level in the body, and are vital to maintaining healthy cells, tissues and organs. There are two groups of EFAs: linoleic acid (LA or omega-6) and alpha-linolenic (LNA or omega-3) acid. EFAs are not created by the body, so we have to ensure that we get enough of them through diet or supplementation. Studies show that most Western diets are lacking in omega-3, which comes from fish; salmon, mackerel, rainbow trout, sardines and eel contain large quantities. The richest vegetarian sources of omega-3 are linseed (flaxseed) oil, which is more than half omega-3, followed by chia and kukui (candlenut) oils, hempseed oil, pumpkin seed oil and canola oil; walnuts, wheatgerm and soya oils also contain small amounts, as do dark green leaves.

Sunflower and safflower are the richest sources of linoleic acid (omega-6), which is also found in flax, hemp, pumpkin, sesame, soybean and walnut. Hempseed oil is the best balanced plant source of both LA and LNA.

The method by which EFA-rich oils are produced is of crucial importance because ingredients central to their function in the body are easily destroyed by light, heat and oxygen. EFAs should never be used for frying, because this converts them into toxins. See entry for Udo's oil.

Essiac Tea

Essiac tea was formulated by Canadian nurse Rene Caisse (essiac is Caisse spelt backwards) in the 1920s. The original formula contains sheep sorrel, Indian rhubarb, burdock and slippery elm. Essiac tea is invaluable in the treatment of any immune system disorder, such as ME, and in the healthy strengthens resistance to infections, and detoxifies the liver and blood. If you take Essiac tea, ensure that your consumption of water is sufficient to remove the waste produced by the detoxifying process the herbs stimulate.

Eucalyptus

The oil of the eucalyptus is probably one of nature's most powerful antiseptics. The rapidly growing tree, a native of Australia and Tasmania and known colloquially as the Australian Fever Tree, has been cultivated in many temperate regions of the world with a view to preventing malarial fevers. Eucalyptus oil is made from the leaves of the tree and is used in respiratory ailments such as coughs, bronchitis and asthma.

Evening Primrose

This is one of the oldest plant-based remedies and a rich source of gammalinolenic acid (GLA). The health benefits to be had from evening primrose oil derive from these GLAs, which iron out the hormonal swings associated with the menstrual cycle. Evening primrose oil needs to be taken in conjunction with Vitamin E, which is essential to stop the oil oxidizing; some EPO products include this vitamin in their formulation.

Fats

Saturated fats – found in, for example, butter, hard cheese, coconut oil and fatty meat products – we can do without because the body can make its own from carbohydrates, proteins or alcohol. These fats generally undermine our health, increasing the risk of cancer and heart disease, and encouraging fluid retention in women before their periods and tooth decay. The fats used in many processed foods – such as margarine, industrially hardened lard, factory-made biscuits, cakes and crisps are particularly harmful. They have been stripped of the essential nutrients (their mineral and vitamin content, as well as their proteins and fibre) present in their parent oil and their formerly beneficial molecular structure changed to inhibit good health. Unsaturated fats – found in, for example, avocado, nuts, olive oil, most vegetable oils, oily fish and fish oils – can not be made by the body and are thus classified as 'essential'; see entry for Essential Fatty Acids.

Fennel

Fennel seed has been used since the time of the ancient Greeks to aid digestion. Fennel tea helps to ease a range of digestive problems, including wind and bloating. However, it should not be taken by pregnant women in whom it may encourage menstruation.

Feverfew (Tanacetum parthenium)

Feverfew is anti-inflammatory, relaxant, vasodilatory (dilates blood vessels) and it stimulates the digestion. It is particularly useful for migraine sufferers as a preventative treatment. Clinical studies have shown it to be effective in reducing the intensity and frequency of attacks in 70 per cent of migraine sufferers. Fever and arthritis are other indications for its use.

Fibre

The fibre or roughage of the diet, such as cereals, nuts and fruits, helps to keep the colon clear but may not remove toxic residue. There is another type of fibre which does assist in the removal of sticky mucus, toxins and hardened matter. One of the best-known is psyllium, or more precisely the husks of this plantain. However, in some people this causes bloating and discomfort. The gentlest fibre I have found is Oligo-fibre, which contains ginger extract and agents which help digest undigested proteins and unfriendly gut bacteria and encourage the growth of *Bifidobacterium bifidus*. The liquid fibre Fructo-litre contains fructooligosaccharides (FOS), one of a group of compounds found in raw fruits and vegetables (such as artichoke, chicory and dandelion) and assists the growth of beneficial gut flora.

Fructo-lite – see Fibre

Garlic

Garlic contains a substance called allicin, which is anti-viral, anti-fungal, antioxidant and anti-bacterial, and is rich in amino acids. These properties make it a natural cleansing agent, capable of breaking down toxins in the bloodstream, fighting yeast organisms and increasing the circulation. It is thought that garlic protects against stomach cancer by preventing the conversion of nitrites and nitrates – substances found in many preserved foods – into cancer-inducing agents called nitrosamines.

Garlic is beneficial for every conceivable ailment and should be included in the diet as a matter of course, raw, cooked or taken in capsule form. It is excellent for immune system disorders.

Ginger

Ginger is very similar to garlic in its purifying action. In Chinese medicine root ginger has been used for centuries to help improve circulation and digestion. Like garlic, it is a wonderful internal cleanser and soother of the gastrointestinal tract.

Glucosamine Sulphate

Glucosamine is a naturally-occurring substance found in high concentrations in the joints. In many arthritis sufferers the ability to produce glucosamine is reduced. Unlike aspirin and other non-steroidal anti-inflammatory drugs (NSAIDs) which, clinical studies have shown, suppress the symptoms of arthritis while accelerating its progress, glucosamine stimulates the production of cartilage and sulphur. (Sulphur is one of the six major elements required by the human body. It maintains elasticity in body tissues.)

Glutamine

Amino acids, such as glutamine, are the building blocks of protein and ensure that maximum absorption is obtained from food. They can switch polarity in the bloodstream, causing the pH to shift towards acidity or alkalinity. Glutamine is the main fuel of the digestive lining, the immune system and, apart from glucose, the only substance that can be used as fuel by the brain.

The product L-Glutamine comes in powder and capsule forms. The powder form is better because it does not irritate even the most delicate system whereas the capsules sometimes do. Glutamine is sensitive to heat and acidity and should not be taken with hot or acidic drinks.

Gluten

It is wise to limit your intake of any foods containing gluten, which can damage the villi lining the small intestine, inhibiting the absorption of nutrients. Wheat is the most glutinous of all grains and is found in a wide range of everyday foods from biscuits and cakes to pasta. Wheatgerm and oatbran contain small amounts of gluten. Sourdoughing wholewheat flour reduces the presence of gluten further, rendering it less gas-forming and easier to digest. Bread made from gluten-free flours is even easier on the digestion.

Grapefruit

Grapefruit seed extract is an antibiotic, anti-fungal and antiviral. It is particularly effective in candidal, bacterial, parasitic and other intestinal disorders and kills infections without laying waste to the good bacteria in the gut.

Grapes

Grape juice sustained the Indian nationalist leader Mahatma Ghandi during his lengthy fasts in protest at British rule. Grapes are an all-round food, nutritious, cleansing and curative. The disorders they help include fatigue, rheumatism and gout, stress, anaemia, and urinary and skin problems (see Refreshing the System on page 124).

Green Energy

If you are not eating organic foods or suspect that you are not getting enough trace elements, supplement your diet with Green Energy foods such as barley grass, wheatgrass, or the algaes (see page 124) chlorella or spirulina.

Green Tea

Japanese or Chinese green tea is lower in tannin and caffeine than ordinary black tea. It also contains antioxidants (see page 25) which help the body to keep healthy.

Hawthorn – see Crataegus

Hypericum (St John's Wort)

The flowering herb St John's Wort has been found to have a success rate with depression comparable to that of Prozac, but without the side-effects associated with that drug's use. Hypericum works by inhibiting or increasing as appropriate the activities of some of the body's own chemicals to maintain fully effective immune responses, and to promote the body's ability to manage stress – for example, by improving the ability to dream during sleep.

Joint Nutrition

Specially designed for people with joint problems, this contains amino acids which make the system more alkaline and ease stiffness. The gentle action of Joint Nutrition works without upsetting the stomach, which in people with illnessess such as arthritis and rheumatism is particularly weak.

Kava-Kava

This member of the pepper family has been used as a relaxant in the South Pacific for centuries. The main constituents of kava-kava – kava lactones – have a sedative action comparable in effectiveness to benzodiazapines, such as valium, but are safe and non-addictive. In addition to aiding quality sleep, kava-kava is helpful in alleviating depression and anxiety. The remedy has a cumulative effect and its benefits may not be felt in some individuals for several days.

Lemon

The lemon contains twice as much Vitamin C as the orange and is rich in bioflavonoids (substances which support the protective action of Vitamin C, are anti-inflammatory, and strengthen the blood vessels). The acids in lemon are transformed into potassium carbonate during digestion. This agent makes the system more alkaline by neutralizing excessive acidity. In addition, the juice of the lemon protects the lining of the digestive tract.

If you have ulcers or a very acidic stomach, try the lemon and olive oil drink (see page 151 for recipe) first. Begin by taking just a teaspoon and slowly, in stages, increase the amount. Only once your system can happily accept the full lemon and olive drink, should you try lemon in water.

Linseed

Soaked linseed is used as a bulking agent or glider to assist the passage of waste through the system. If the linseed is not soaked it will stick to the gut and cause irritation by pulling mucous from the gut lining.

Note: Soaked linseed has a totally different function from that of linseed oil (see Essential Fatty Acids on page 131).

Lipo-Plex

This supplement – designed for people with joint problems – includes fish oil concentrates, coenzyme Q10, olive oil and vitamins C and E. It is an ideal substitute for Udo's oil (see page 144) for busy people or those who travel a great deal.

Magnesium

Magnesium is vital to the proper functioning of the nervous system. It aids the alkaline-acid balance in the gut and the absorption of calcium. Shortfalls in its intake have been linked to diabetes, high blood pressure, heart disease and problems in pregnancy. Low intake of magnesium is also believed to be a contributory factor in osteoporosis and to heighten the effects of PMS (see Cal-M on page 127).

Milk

Cow's milk is very difficult for humans to digest and what is not digested stays in the system, blocking the lungs and the lymphatic system as mucous. All of us have an intolerance to milk, but whereas most of us get away with it some people, such as asthmatics and those lacking in the enzyme lactase, do not and have to throw off the overflow of toxins through the lungs. In sensitive children, cow's milk can destroy the stomach lining. The proteins in goat's milk are closer to those in human milk and thus easier for us to digest than cow's protein. Intolerance to cow's milk is exacerbated by a lack of unsaturated oils, such as linseed or Udo's oil (see page 144).

Milk Thistle (Silybum marianum)

Noted for its good effect on a sluggish liver, milk thistle inhibits free radicals and stimulates the synthesis of protein to replace damaged liver cells with new ones. Milk thistle is a rich source of the detoxifier and antioxidant silymarin.

Caution: A large dose can lead to a healing crisis and have a slight laxative effect.

Millet

High in protein and low in starches, this highly nutritious cereal is – unlike most starches – easy to digest. It contains all eight essential amino acids and is the only grain that is a complete protein and alkali-forming. Millet is high in the mineral salt silicon (an element of collagen), which helps to keep mind and body together and functioning well.

Missing Link

The Missing Link is a super-food product formulated entirely from wholefoods and food concentrates. It contains the eight factors we need every day: friendly bacteria, soluble and insoluble dietary fibre, the EFAs omega-3 and omega-6, digestive enzymes, balanced protein, vitamins, major and trace minerals, and phytochemicals (molecules from health-giving plants). These are included in the form of flax seed, sunflower seed, blackstrap molasses, rice bran, nutritional yeast, alfalfa, carrot, apple, hesperidin, sesame seed, liquorice root, sprouted green barley, spirulina (blue/green algae), nettle, broccoli powder, cherry powder, parsley, kelp, vanilla bean, ginger root, sage, rosemary, yucca and garlic.

Missing Link is added to food after cooking. It can be mixed with vegetable juice or yoghurt, or sprinkled on salads or cereals. The suggested dose is 2–3 tablespoons each day. However, this will not be right for everybody so, if you take it, start with one teaspoon each day and gradually increase the dosage. One half of a tablespoon once or twice a day is usually sufficient. A headache or bad skin will tell you if the dosage is too high. After taking Missing Link for a couple of months your skin should feel the benefits.

MSM

Methylsulphonylmethane provides the body with sulphur, a component of protein structure and one of the six major elements required by the human body to function properly. MSM is found in the body tissues and fluids but its presence diminishes with age. Sulphur is on continuous call by the body to strengthen and stabilize structural integrity, as a vital constituent in connective tissue, and to keep hair, skin and nails healthy. Without the correct amounts of sulphur new tissue cells become rigid, causing pain and inflammation. I use MSM in cases of joint problem, such as arthritis, to ease discomfort and maintain tissue elasticity.

Mullein (Verbascum thapsus)

Mullein has for centuries been used successfully as a remedy for all lung diseases in both animals and humans. In Ireland it used to be cultivated in gardens because of its demand as a remedy for pulmonary consumption. Mullein is of value as a remedy for piles and other inflammation of the mucuous membranes as well as diarrhoea and frostbite. For asthmatics a blend of mullein tea is helpful.

Nettle

The stinging nettle plant contains a host of invaluable minerals, including iron, phospherous, potassium and calcium. If you fancy harvesting your own, pick them in spring when the leaves are young and tender. Avoid nettles growing by the side of the road – these are more likely to have been sprayed. Once you have selected your nettles, wash them very carefully, then cook them as you would spinach.

Papaya (Pawpaw)

Papaya is a good source of Vitamin C and beta-carotene and because it contains papain, an enzyme similar to pepsin in that it breaks down proteins, it is easily digestible. It is the premier fruit in cases of infection or if the gut lining is in need of repair.

Pilates Method

The principles of this method were devised by the late Joseph H. Pilates some 60 years ago. The method aims to improve muscle control, flexibility, strength, coordination and tone through the execution of precise movements with specific breathing patterns. It teaches breath control and body awareness, it improves posture and relieves back pain. The method is appropriate for all ages and levels of fitness and is recommended by osteopaths and physiotherapists. Many of my clients have benefited from the Pilates method and enhanced their overall level of health by incorporating it into their routine.

Probiotics

The practice of using beneficial bacteria to restore balance to the digestive system is called probiotics. Various probiotic supplements are available. No two people have the same digestive system and what is appropriate for one person will not be right for the next, so when first using products such as Acidophilus always err on the side of caution. Start with a mild milk-free model suitable for children – *Bifidobacterium infantis* – and take less than the recommended dosage. This model is also appropriate for people with what I regard as advanced degenerative illnesses, such as asthma, panic attacks or high blood pressure. One strength up from *Bifidobacterium infantis* is a model which combines *Lactobacillus acidophilus* and *Bifidobacterium bifidum*. There are stronger models still, but before taking them it is wise to consult a professional therapist or chemist to ensure that they are appropriate for you.

Pulses

These are wonderful if they are allowed to sprout before they are cooked. By taking pulses on this stage further, you make them less starchy, easier to cook and to digest – and they taste better.

To slightly sprout pulses: soak them (giving them double the time recommended on the bag or packet), rinse them, then remove them to a glass jar topped with muslin where they have air and can be kept moist; rinse them every day to prevent them drying out. They should start to peep out after two or three days. If you are sprouting larger beans, watch them carefully because they tend to rot more easily than smaller types.

Once the beans have sprouted, cook them to perfection, eat them in small amounts and chew them very thoroughly. As far as the digestion is concerned, soya beans are an easier pre-fermented alternative to pulses.

Q10

This coenzyme (also called ubiquinone or Vitamin Q) is a circulation-boosting antioxidant which plays a central role in the energy production of cells. A deficiency in ubiquinone can lead to heart failure, fatigue and gum disease.

Quinoa

A small easily digestible rice-like seed from South America, quinoa contains more protein than other starches. Quinoa pasta is also available, providing an alternative to wheat pasta.

Reckeweg, Dr

Hans Heinrich Reckeweg was a German homeopath who founded a company with the purpose of manufacturing his own complex homeopathic formulas. The Reckweg complexes given as remedies in this book are very mild and I have no hesitation in recommending them for use without medical supervision. They are obtainable from high quality homeopathic chemists.

Rescue Remedy

This is a combination of five of the Bach flower remedies created by Harley Street physician Dr Edward Bach in the 1930s. These are: rock rose (for terror), impatiens (for impatience), clematis (for dreaminess and lack of interest in the here and now), star of Bethlehem (for the after-effects of shock) and cherry plum (for fear of mental breakdown).

Rice

Normal rice is a starch. Protein is obtainable from the pre-fermented rice eaten in Japan and southern India and thus is a good source of protein for vegetarians. Do not eat polished (white) rice. This has been denuded of the grain's essential health-giving properties, specifically the B vitamin thiamin. Boiled brown rice is soothing to the digestive system and an age-old cure for diarrhoea.

Sage

Sage has been used for innumerable health problems from diseases of the liver and kidneys to asthma, ulcers and snake bites. It is particularly valued as a tonic – taken in the form of a tea or infusion – in cases of nervous exhaustion and weakness of the stomach or digestion. Sage also forms the basis of some remedies for menopause-related problems.

St John's Wort – see Hypericum

Salt

A high intake of salt (sodium) is linked to high blood pressure and heart disease, and also has the effect of flushing calcium from the body.

Salt encourages the body to produce insulin by faciliating glucose absorption and can thus bring on a craving for sugar and lead to other symptoms of hypoglycaemia, such as increased appetite.

Sauerkraut

The word means sour (pickled) cabbage. Sauerkraut is made by mixing finely shredded cabbage with sea salt and spices, organizing the mixture into tightly packed layers and leaving it to ferment. This process produces lactic acid which, when ingested, kills off unfriendly or putrefactive bacteria in the gut. As well as being a great system cleanser, Sauerkraut is a rich source of Vitamin C, calcium and potassium.

Seaweed – see Algae

Selenium

Selenium is a trace element which forms part of an enzyme that protects cells against free radicals (see page 25). The paucity of the trace element in the agricultural land of Northern Europe is reflected in the low selenium content of the average Northern European's diet – estimated at about 45 micrograms (the intake recommended by the World Health Organization is 50 to 200 mcg). Relatively high levels of selenium are to be found in fish, liver, kidneys and cereals.

Shou Wu Chih

The main constituents of this Chinese herbal tonic are polygonum multiflorum thunb., angelica sinensis and polygonatum chinense. Shou Wu Chih has the effect of raising the body's energy levels and is an excellent pick-me-up for people of all ages and sexes in cases of debility, neuresthenia, anaemia, general weakness and convalescence.

Silymarin (croisia) – see Milk Thistle

Slippery Elm (Ulmus fulva)

The substance obtained from the inner bark of the slippery elm plant is soothing, healing and highly nutritious. Powdered slippery elm can be taken in many instances where the digestive system will tolerate no other food. It is also available as a tea, blended with marshmallow root. In this form slippery elm soothes the digestion, and helps stomach disorders and diarrhoea. In addition to its internal uses, slippery elm may also be applied externally as a poultice for wounds, ulcers, boils and burns.

Soya

Soya beans and the products made from them, such as miso and tofu, are high in protein, iron, calcium, B-compex vitamins and lecithin (a substance which keeps cholesterol levels in the blood low). However, because soya contains a thyroid-depressing element, it is advisable to eat small amounts and to balance your intake – as the Japanese do – by eating iodine-rich algae foods such as seaweed.

Spelt

An ancient variety of wheat, spelt (also called farro) does not ferment and although it contains gluten it is digestible by people with allergies who can not eat ordinary wheat flour or grains such as rye or barley. Spelt-pasta and spelt-bread are also available.

Spirulina– see Algae

Sugar

The first point that needs to be made about sugar is that it is not essential. We do not need it to give us energy. Fruits and vegetables are just two of the food types that are broken down into sugar by the process of digestion. In fact, sugar saps our energy and depletes our resources. Any food that increases the glucose levels quickly – as sugar does – produces the double effect of increasing acidity and reducing the body's absorption of calcium. It is reckoned that consuming 100g of sugar (equivalent to a 5oz bar of chocolate or a can of soda) can suppresss the immune system for about six hours.

Sugar promotes the secretion of insulin. This suppresses the formation of ketoacids – which help clear excess sodium and water from the kidneys – and increases the excretion of magnesium in the urine. Even slight magnesium deficiency is thought to cause emotional upsets, such as irritability, anxiety and depression. Sugar also consumes calcium – in the young this leads to cavities, and in the old to brittle bone disease and osteoporosis – and hampers the action of neutrophils, which protect the body against invading microorganisms.

Artificial sweeteners trigger the same response as sugar and increase the level of insulin in the body. Soft drinks such as Diet Coke – which are virtually sugared water – work in much the same way and are similarly addictive.

Thyme

Thyme boosts the immune system, protects against viral and bacterial infections and stimulates the nervous system. Taken as a tea, thyme is useful in cases of wind and gastric disorders. Used as an oil and added to a warm bath, thyme strengthens and soothes the nerves.

Udo's Oil

Geneticist, biochemist and nutritionist, Udo Erasmus developed his Udo's Choice Ultimate Oil Blend to address the need for a single oil that provides both omega-3 and omega-6 in the correct amounts. Too much of one EFA (see entry above) will cause a deficiency in the other. The correct ratio, according to Erasmus, is 2:1 of 3s to 6s. Udo's oil contains oils from fresh, certified organic flax, sesame and sesame seeds, as well as oils from wheatgerm, ricegerm and oatgerm.

Umeboshi Plum

An Umeboshi plum a day keeps the haemorrhoids away. Umeboshi plums are produced by pickling Ume plums (exceptional among fruits for their nutritional content) with sea salt and shiso leaves. They cleanse the system by changing the acidity in the gut.

Valerian

This plant has a powerful effect on the nervous systems of many animals, such as cats, as well as humans. Legend has it that the attraction of rats to the Pied Piper of Hamelin was due to the valerian he carried with him. The herb's soothing effect on the mind and nervous system make it of especial benefit to those suffering from stress, over-work or insomnia.

Verbena/ Vervain

Several species of this family are used in herbal medicines. Vervain (*Verbena officinalis*) is prescribed for insomnia, as a diuretic, for wounds and to stop diarrhoea. Lemon verbena is used as a sedative and to reduce fever. Verbena also helps in cases of dyspepsia, indigestion and wind.

Techniques and Recipes

THE pH TEST

I have included this test just for a bit of fun to enable you to see where you are on the pH scale. A pH test will tell you how alkaline or acid your body is. Low pH values indicate acidity, high pH values alkalinity (see page 24). Saliva and urine are measured on a scale of 0 to 14. A neutral pH is around 7. The value you should be aiming for is given below. Whereas it is generally better to have saliva that is slightly more alkaline than acid, the reverse is true of urine. As we have already seen the balance in the various parts of the digestive system changes depending on the chemical response, and this is reflected in the pH values of our saliva and urine (see page 24).

The pH profile of most of the people I have come across during the course of my work tends to be acid saliva and urine. Rebalancing the pH is very straightforward – just follow the three Rs of health: volume, thorough chewing and always giving your particular system what it can digest, with or without help.

The Values

Normal early morning pH patterns for saliva and urine are 6.2 to 6.4 and 5.5 to 6.0 respectively. After the first urine test, the second reading for both urine and saliva should be 6.4. A first urine value of over 6.2 indicates too much alkalinity. Someone with this reading is likely to wake up feeling tired from too many waste products building up in the blood.

Danger Values

These are saliva below 6.0 (too acid), and urine above 6.8 (too alkaline). Acid saliva pH and alkaline urine pH indicate several negative points about the system – a congested and toxic liver, adrenal exhaustion, digestive problems, acid blood and lymph, and an inability to absorb esssential fatty acids.

How to test

You can buy pH tape or testing strips for saliva and urine from chemists and health food shops. Most of these kits involve placing the saliva in a spoon – or the urine in some other receptacle – and then dipping about a one-inch piece of paper torn from a strip in the solution. You compare the reading to the colour chart provided with the strip. Ensure that the reading is done about 4 to 6 seconds after dipping the strip in the solution.

Saliva tends to be more stable than urine and thus provides a more accurate pH reading. However, like body temperature, pH values of both saliva and urine fluctuate throughout the day. The best time to test both of them – and especially urine – is in the morning before breakfast. Always drink a glass of water before testing at this time and wait a few minutes before carrying out the test. If an early morning test is not possible, complete only the saliva test and carry this out either before eating or two hours after eating – testing immediately after food will automatically produce a higher reading.

BOOSTING THE IMMUNE SYSTEM

Skin brushing and cold water bathing work on the same principle of increasing circulation to boost the immune system and stimulating the lymphatic. They are very effective methods of keeping the body feeling well toned. You can use them together (i.e. skin brushing followed by a cold dip) or separately.

Skin Brushing

Skin brushing stimulates both the circulation and the lymphatic drainage system. It is a worthwhile technique to learn and to use whenever you take a bath or shower. Regular brushing improves the texture of skin and, more importantly, keeps the pores clear so that toxins can be expelled through them. Clogged skin pores can put pressure on the body's other eliminatory organs, such as the liver, kidneys and bowels.

First, choose your implement. A long-handled wooden bristle brush is, I think, the most efficient; alternatives are a hand-mitt or brush or a loofah. You should find the tingling sensation produced by skin brushing pleasurable. However, if the brush is too harsh for your liking, soak it in warm water overnight to soften the bristles.

Brush with long, firm strokes in the direction of the heart, starting with the backs of the hands, then the palms, and working up the arms, inner and outer. Do the legs next, starting with the feet. Include some circular movements over the outer thighs and buttocks and in towards the inner thighs where the lymph nodes are situated. Adopt a clockwise motion over the abdomen. Brush the lower back and the sides of the body. Stop when you reach a point level with the heart, then begin to work downwards, starting with the neck and shoulders. Lastly, brush each armpit, in the direction of your breast.

Brushing is best done before a bath or shower, so that the dead skin and dirt are washed away rather than remain clinging to your body. Try to skin-brush every day for the first two weeks, then cut it back to a few days a week, varying the days.

Do not brush broken, inflamed or infected skin or near varicose veins or patches of eczema or psoriasis.

Cold Bathing

The originator of cold-water bathing was the German Sebastian Kneipp whose therapy is widely practised in his homeland and beyond. It forms part of my daily regime because it is the best self-help stimulation of the lymphatic system available.

The best time for a cold bath is early in the morning when the body is at its most relaxed. A cold water dip triggers the sympathetic nervous system, stimulating respiration, heartbeat, raising the blood sugar and increasing the production of the white blood cells which fight infection. A cold bath has the same effect for the whole body as putting ice on an injury – it increases the circulation and thus the body's resistance

It is wise to get your body used to cold water bathing in stages. Do not be a martyr and spend ages perishing with cold. Start by spending just a minute or two in the water, which should be just cold enough to give you goosepimples. Ensure that your feet have adapted to the temperature before lowering your body into the water. The body should be immersed in the water up to and including the neck. Over a period of two or three months the time you spend in the water can be increased to 20 minutes, and the temperature lowered from 20 to 16 degrees Celsius.

Once out of the bath and towelled dry, do not try to reheat the body quickly. This will happen of its own accord, as the body reacts to the cold water. If it takes you longer than half an hour to forty-five minutes to get warm after bathing, you have spent too long in the water.

REFRESHING THE SYSTEM

History gives us numerous examples of clearing the system periodically as part of the ongoing process of life. In the Bible, for example, there is a reference to cleaning vessels and cleansing the colon. We should try to look at it in the same way, as natural as taking a bath or having a hair cut. Each culture has at one time developed its own method of cleansing, derived from foods. In Persia a type of fermented goat's milk, called Kushi is used; in Germany Sauerkraut juice performs the same function, and in Japan plums from the Umeboshi plant.

A balance between mind, body and spirit enables us to progress and to achieve in the purest sense. Throughout history artists have understood this and been aware of the intimate connection between their creativity and their spiritual growth. Michelangelo, for example, would not start a major painting without having a 20-day fast beforehand. Cleansing through diet is also a central plank of the yogi's path to spiritual development. For those of us with less lofty aspirations, a cleansed body makes life far easier and a great deal more enjoyable.

It is important to make a distinction between fasting and starving. The complete absence of food is damaging to the body. The idea that the intestines need a complete rest from food in order to repair themselves is erroneous. The mucosal cells lining the intestines rely on food to keep them healthy. If they become eroded by the withholding of food, they are less able to protect us against bacteria permeating the lining and gaining access to adjacent tissues and, eventually, to the bloodstream.

Which System?

Some cleansing programmes are so drastic that they can strip the gut and make it bleed. Fasting, too, is not advisable for those who are working and have low blood sugar (see page 102). It strains the body unnecessarily and risks waking up with an angry start substances that should be moved out of the system quietly. During the fast there is a danger of the blood sugar dropping and toxins reaching the brain. Just as it is not advisable to use a sport to get fit, so it is not a good idea to fast in order to cleanse. Your body must already be in good shape if it is to derive any benefit from fasting. If you want to try it, do not undertake it alone but go to a clinic or health centre where you will be under professional supervision.

Regime

Autumn is a good time to clear the body. It will make your immune system stronger and more resilient over the winter period. The system of cleansing I use – which is very gentle – consists of organic grapes (black or white varieties, but not seedless), garlic (take this in capsule form if you are worried about your popularity) and lots of water. This regime rids the body of stress and gives it a chance to heal. There is a list of 'must dos'. These are:

- Do not eat pounds of grapes. If you do, you will explode. Use the hand-size rule (see page 31) for each modest meal. Have four or five of these meals throughout the day. This will ensure that the blood sugar remains even.
- The grapes must be chewed perfectly, including the pips, which contain beneficial oils. This will really test your resolve – although easy to digest, grapes taste very bitter when they are well chewed.
- Drink 4–5 litres (7–9 pints) of water a day. It is important not to drink less than the minimum. The toxins the diet will be releasing must be flushed through the system and not allowed to wreak havoc within it.

An alternative to grapes is fresh figs, a favoured cleansing food of the Greeks. Like grapes, they make the digestive system alkaline. If you prefer this option, the stipulation about the amount of water that must be drunk is the same.

Chewed very well and slowly neither of these foods should produce a drama, so do not be put off by the worry that you might be forced to spend days in the lavatory.

It takes the body three days to realize that something is happening, so if you want to clear out the body you need to devote at least this number of days to the regime. Five or six days is ideal. At the end of it you should feel refreshed and energized.

It is a good idea to have an ongoing programme of periodically resting the body. One way of unloading a little as you go is to rest the digestion one day a week by eating only vegetables. Every little bit helps.

Nettle was once a favourite spring cleanser. The nutritious young leaves, which taste like spinach and are full of selenium and other trace elements, were picked and cooked as a vegetable or made into soup. Nettle tea is widely available and very therapeutic.

(See entry for Grapes in Chapter Six, Foods, Supplements and Remedies.)

Whole Lemon And Olive Oil Drink

Lemon combined with olive oil counteracts acidity in the stomach, making the system more alkaline, and clears undigested food particles.

Ingredients:

1 medium lemon, preferably organic
1 tablespoon of cold pressed extra Virgin olive oil
300–450 ml (1/2–3/4 pint) of orange or other juice, or water

Cut the lemon into quarters, retaining the rind and pips. Place in a blender. Add the juice or water, then the olive oil. Blend at high speed for two minutes. Strain the mixture to separate the juice from the pulp.

The juice may be drunk in one go or taken in two or three separate portions during the day.

Acknowledgements

My thanks to Fiona MacIntyre at Ebury for her belief in this project, to my editor at Ebury, Joanna Sheehan, for all her patience, to Ian McLellan, my agent, for his support and humour and to Tessa Rose for being the perfect writing partner. And to Cath who can calm any storms with her Celtic humour.

I would also like to thank Dr Schellander of the Liongate Clinic, 8 Chilston Road, Tonbridge Wells, Kent; Roger Wilson of Biopathica; Lennart Sedergard and all at Noma Complex Homeopathy.

Finally, I would like to thank the following for their help in providing information: Ian of Savant Distribution Limited, Leeds; Penny Davenport of The Nutrition Line, Burwash Common, East Sussex; Liz Scott of G & G Foods, East Grinstead, West Sussex; Pilates Studio/Danceworks, London W1; and IMT Technologies Limited, University of Birmingham, Edgbaston, Birmingham

Resources

The following practitioners are highly recommended by the author. Gudrun Jonsson has been treated by them all and has benefited enormously from their individual talents, helping her to maintain good health. She often refers her patients to them when appropriate:

1) **Dr Fritz Schellander MD (Vienna), L.M.S.S.A. (London) and a member of the British Holistic Medical Association**
A general practitioner for many years, Dr Schellander now combines oxygen and chelation treatments which many have found invaluable on their path to better health. For further information, call 01892 543535.

2) **Gerry Gajadharsing DO MRO, Registered Osteopath**
An experienced osteopath, his treatment is geared to the individual and he complements his treatments with stress management techniques. He has successfully treated both adults and children, who have been referred to him by the author, for a variety of symptoms and conditions. For further information, call 020 7487 4204.

3) **Peta Knaggs**
Peta Knaggs has been a bodyworker for six years and specializes in body harmony which she has pioneered in a purpose built pool – an exquisite healing experience benefiting many clients. For further information, call 020 7486 1711.

4) **Dr Franklin's Panchakarma Institute & Research Centre,** Chowara P.O., Thiruvananthapuram. Kerala, S. India. Pin-695 501. Tel: 0091-471-480870, Fax: 0091-471-482870

5) **The Natural Mineral Water Information Service** publishes a free booklet, Body Thoughts, about the benefits of drinking water. For a copy send a stamped self-addressed DL envelope to: Natural Mineral Water Information Service, PO Box 6, Hampton, Middlesex TW12 2HH. For further information from the Natural Mineral Water Information Service visit the website:
http://www.naturalmineralwater.org.

6) **Bodydoctor fitness**
David Marshall is the fitness expert who I work with and he keeps us all in shape. For information, tel: 020 7586 6222 or visit his website on: www.bodydoctorfitness.com Email: david@bodydoctorfitness.com.

7) **Swaddles Green Farm** produce a variety of high quality organic fresh meats and stocks as well as a wide range of other products including ready-prepared meals. For information, call 01460 234387 or fax 01460 234591.

To find out more about Gudrun's London practice or the products she recommends, you can find us on the worldwide website at:
http://www.gudrunjonsson.com
or
gudrunsproducts@legado.co.uk
or write to us enclosing an s.a.e. at: 2 Napier Road, London W14 8LQ, England

Note: Most of the products mentioned in this book are available by mail order or in person from H. Lloyd Chemist at 1 Russell Gardens, London W14 8EZ, tel: 020 7603 4761. The Powerbreathe is available direct from IMT Technologies Limited, Sports, Medicine and Human Performance Unit, University of Birmingham.

Further Reading

Dries, Jan and Inge, *The Complete Book of Food Combining* (Element)
Hay, Louise L., *You Can Heal Your Life* (Eden Grove)
Johnson, L.R., edited by, *Physiology of the Gastrointestinal Tract* (Raven Press)
Stamp, Terence & Buxton, Elizabeth, *The Stamp Collection Cookbook* (Ebury Press)

Index

absorption 20–1
acid/alkaline balance 23–4, 33–4, 37, 46
acid foods 77
acid-forming foods 46, 52, 61–2, 70–1, 78–9, 83, 94, 98, 101, 113, 118–19, 122
acidity 51–2, 82, 100–1, 136
  low 22–3
Acidophilus 40, 56, 82, 98–9, 119, 122, 123, 140
acupuncture 73, 99, 117
adrenaline 29, 30, 55, 58, 86, 111, 114
alcohol 20, 25, 54, 57, 65, 82, 88, 91, 103, 114–15, 122
alfalfa 87
algae 124, 143
alkali-forming foods 61–2, 110, 117
aloe vera 40, 76, 77–8, 119–20, 122, 125
amino acids 20
angelica 99, 125
anger 40, 86
aniseed 72, 76, 79, 125
antibiotics 39, 47, 78, 100, 108–9, 117
anti-depressants 15
anti-fungal foods 79
antioxidants 15, 25, 126, 135
anxiety 40, 76, 87–8, 95, 114, 136, 143
apple 76, 112, 119, 125–6
aromatherapy 99, 108, 113, 117, 122
arteriosclerosis 25
arthritis 12, 23, 25, 35, 49, 58, 100–1, 126, 129, 133, 134, 136, 138
asthma 22, 23, 36, 47, 49, 70–3, 132, 139, 140
atherosclerosis 89
auto-immune disorders 22, 108, 125
avocado 37, 77

baby formulas 72
Bach's Rescue Remedy 88, 141
backache 36
bacteria, *see* microflora
barley 126
Basic Programme 55, 66
bathing 74, 86
  cold 106, 110, 148–9
  salt 96, 119
beetroot 77–8
beta-carotene 126
Bifidobacterium 72, 102, 133,140
bile 19–20, 23, 75, 77, 129
BioCarbonate 123
bioflavonoids 136
biopathy 11
biscuits 51, 107
bitters 80
bloating 50–1, 99, 100, 116, 133
blood cells, white 14–15
blood pressure, high 36, 86–9, 103, 137, 140, 141
blood sugar, *see* hypoglycaemia
body shape 37, 63
Boswellia 82, 126
bowel disease 75
bowel movements 56, 58
brain, lower 14–16, 115
bran 54, 55–6
bread 35, 46, 70, 79, 107, 115, 119, 120–1, 135
breakfast 30, 51, 55–6, 106, 112, 123, 125

breast-feeding 72
breathing 73, 78
breathing machine 116, 126–7

caffeine 103
calcium 18, 20, 21, 96, 127, 143
Cal-M 40, 71, 82, 83, 85, 88, 91, 96, 102, 113, 116, 123, 127
calories 36–7
cancer 12, 25, 49, 126, 132
  stomach 22, 120, 133
Candida 23
Candistatin 76, 127, 131
carbohydrate 19, 21, 23, 51, 101, 107
cataracts 25
catarrh 73–4, 125
cellulose 21
cereals 51, 53, 71, 133, 137
cerebral haemorrhage 25
chamomile 99, 113, 122, 128
change 63–5
charcoal 80, 128
cheese 35, 37, 85, 90, 113, 119, 122, 128
chelation 91, 111, 128
chewing 21, 28, 35, 51, 52, 55, 61, 76, 94, 97, 110, 122
chicken 98
children 70, 72, 112
Chinese medicine 40, 134
chlorella 124
chocolate 51, 85, 96, 107, 113, 115, 119
cholesterol, high 89–91
chromium 129
cider vinegar 101, 119, 123, 127, 129
circulation 49, 106, 129, 134, 140, 147
Citrase 127
cleansing programme 149–51
cod liver oil 71, 102
coeliac disease 22
coffee 36, 57, 85, 88, 91, 96, 113, 115, 122
colds 48–9, 74, 125, 130
colitis 15, 49, 97, 99
colon 20
  irrigation 109, 111, 118
constipation 36, 40, 50, 56, 71, 75–8, 104, 107, 112, 118
controllers 75
coronary thrombosis 25
coughs 125, 132
cow's protein 72, 74, 85, 128, 137
cranial osteopathy 78, 79, 86, 102, 113
crateagus 96, 129
Crypts of Lieberkuhn 19
cystitis 46, 49, 78–9, 126

daily regime 55–6
dairy products 70–1, 74, 100
dehydration 35–6
depression 23, 51, 109, 135, 136, 143
dermatitis 22
diabetes 22, 35, 48, 75, 92, 103, 125, 137
diarrhoea 51, 115, 139, 143, 145
diet 32–7
digestive system 13–14, 17–22, 27, 51
digestive problems 48
dill 77, 130
dinner 56, 107, 112–13
diverticulitis 94, 97, 99
drinks 35–6, 56–8, 86, 91, 96
drugs 15, 24, 25
  see also medication
duodenum 19, 22, 77
dysbiosis 48

eating habits 28–33, 55, 57, 76, 87, 94, 112, 115
echinacea 74, 110, 130
eczema 22, 49, 125
eggs 100
elderberry extract 74, 130
elderflower 74, 130
elderly 79, 112
emotions 12, 40
energy 12, 20–1, 30, 49–51, 64, 66, 92
enteric nervous system 14–16
enterocytes 14
Enzyme Aid 98, 130
enzymes 34, 50, 51, 86, 102, 107, 113, 130–1, 138

escapism 43–4
essential fatty acids 90–1, 117, 119, 131, 138, 144
essential oils 72, 74, 113
Essiac tea 110, 131
eucalyptus 72, 74, 132
evening primrose oil 117, 132
exercise 23, 38–9, 56

fasting 149–50
fatigue 23, 36, 48, 126, 135, 140
fats 18–20, 21, 22, 53, 89, 94, 122, 132
  see also oils
fennel 79, 91, 99, 132–3
fermentation 29, 39–40, 46
fermenting foods 94
feverfew 86, 113, 133
fibre 23, 55, 71, 83, 98–9, 129, 133, 138
figs 150
fish 53, 57, 59, 90, 98, 131
fish oil 102, 137
flax oil 117
floatation therapy 73, 102
fluid retention 132
flushers 56, 58
food additives 25, 70
food allergies 22, 23, 45–7
food colourings 70
food combining 53–4, 123
food poisoning 79–81
free radicals 15, 25, 127, 137, 142
freshness of food 34
Fructo-lite 133
fruit 34, 51, 54, 55, 60, 71, 97, 107, 133

gall bladder 19, 22, 77, 126
gall stones 36
garlic 74, 79, 91, 133–4, 150
gastric acids 18, 22–3, 51–2, 76, 79
gastritis 22
genetic blueprint 47–8, 50, 67
ginger 134
  and lemon tea 77, 107, 113
ginseng 87
glucosamine sulphate 102, 134
glutamine 15, 21, 134
  see also L-Glutamine
glutathione 15
gluten 52, 100, 113, 122, 134–5
glycogen 21
gout 81–2, 135
grapefruit 113, 135
grapes 135, 150
grazing 30
Green Energy 40, 56, 69, 106, 113, 135
green tea 135
gut, *see* digestive system

haemorrhoids 82, 130, 139, 144
happiness 42, 43
Hay System, *see* food combining
hayfever 46, 49
headaches 40, 49, 84–6
health 11, 43
heartburn 36
heart disease 12, 40, 103, 129, 132, 137, 141
heavy metals 24
hempseed oil 131
hepatitis 22
herbs 54, 60, 77, 86, 97–8
  infusions 71
  tea 71, 99, 110, 122
homeopathic formulas 69, 141
homeostasis 40
hunger 51
hyperactivity 112
hypericum 88, 115, 135
hypertension, *see* blood pressure, high
hypoglycaemia 30, 37, 44–5, 52, 59, 84, 87, 102–8, 114, 116, 117, 142, 149

illness 11, 17, 43–9
ileum 19
immune system 13, 14, 17–18, 38–9, 103, 108–10, 131, 134, 143, 144, 147–9
immunoglobins 19
impotence 91–3

indigestion 22, 23, 36, 94, 125, 145
inertia 49
infection 15, 135, 139, 144
inflammation 49
influenza 49, 74, 130
insomnia 77, 86, 95–6, 116, 144, 145
insulin 19, 40, 86, 103, 129, 142, 143
iron 18, 21
irritability 86
irritable bowel syndrome 15, 23, 96–100, 118

Japanese food 33
jejenum 19, 20
Joint Nutrition 136
joint problems 36, 100–2, 126, 136, 137, 138

kava-kava 96, 115, 136
kidneys 21, 78–9

L-Glutamine 94, 98–9, 106, 122, 134
lactic acid 100, 142
large intestine 20, 21
late meals 30
laughter 29, 39
leaky gut 17, 46, 108–9
lemon 36, 74, 136
lemon and olive oil 77, 91, 98, 107, 110, 119, 123, 136, 151
life force 92
lifestyle 42, 76
linseed 91, 102, 118, 131, 136
Lipo-Plex 137
liver 15, 19–21, 40, 75, 77, 84, 89, 91, 95, 137
lunch 42, 51, 56, 58–60, 112–13
lungs 70, 139
lymphatic system 17, 23, 25, 39, 74, 147–8
lymphocytes 14

magnesium 91, 96, 127, 137, 143
malabsorption 11, 21–2, 51
massage 39, 73, 82, 86, 88, 99, 108, 117, 122
ME 108–11, 131
meat 53, 57, 81, 83, 88, 90, 98
medication 15, 24, 39–40, 68–9, 89, 96, 121
meditation 39, 42, 96
Mediterranean principle 57
menopause 141
microflora 17–18, 23, 25–6, 39–40, 75, 118, 119, 138
  in babies 72
  overgrowth 22, 23, 34
  probiotics 139–40
middle age 28, 51
migraine 37, 75, 111–13, 133
milk 35, 54, 74, 113, 137
milk thistle 91, 113, 137
millet 137–8
minerals 19, 20–1, 56
  supplements 69, 138
Missing Link 56, 69, 82, 88, 91, 99, 102, 106, 107, 113, 138
mood swings 46, 48
mouth 18, 20, 21
mouth ulcer 23, 120
MSM 102, 138
mucosal lining 14–15
mullein 71, 74, 139

nervous system 14, 137, 144
nettle 123, 139, 151
nitrogen 15, 20
nuts 53, 71, 94, 98, 100, 133

oil 97, 132
  unsaturated 56, 71, 82, 102, 137
Oligo-fibre 77, 133
olive leaf tincture 91
olive oil 71, 98
  see also lemon and olive oil
omega-3/6 oils 90–1, 119, 131, 138, 144
onions 74
orange 85
organic foods 34
osteoarthritis 70
osteopathy 73, 102
osteoporosis 22, 137, 144

over-eating 31–2, 40, 51, 55, 104, 115, 120
over-exercising 100
oxygen therapy, *see* chelation

pancreas 19, 77, 103
panic attacks 40, 114–16, 140
papaya 139
pectin 125–6
pepsin 76
periods, irregular 40
pH 24, 123
  testing 110, 146–7
Pilates method 78, 82, 102, 139
PMS 23, 40, 116–17, 137
pollution 24, 25, 70
potato 35
probiotics 139–40
processed foods 70, 106, 132
progesterone 112
prostaglandins 116, 125
protein 18–19, 20, 21, 23, 53–6, 59, 74, 77, 100, 122
  undigested 81, 83, 90, 97
prunes 56, 77, 107
psoriasis 119, 125
psyllium 133
pulses 35, 140
purgatives 68, 76

Q10 140
quinoa 140

raw foods 34, 35, 99, 122
reactions 68
Reckeweg, Dr 69, 141
refined foods 24, 33, 34, 39, 51, 70, 83
reflexology 73, 79, 82, 84, 88, 99, 108, 113, 117, 122
relaxation 76, 86
  when eating 28–9, 57, 94
rheumatism 49, 100, 125, 135, 136
rice 80, 141

SAD 105
sage 71, 72, 99, 110, 141
salad 54, 59–60
salad dressings 54
saliva 18, 20, 21, 24, 146–7
salt 70, 88, 141–2
  bath 96, 119
Sauerkraut 77–8, 123, 142, 149
seafood 57, 81, 90
seaweed 124, 142
secretin 19
seeds 54
selenium 142, 151
self-persuasion 66
senility 25
sex drive 91–3
shiatsu 88, 99
Shou Wu Chih 110, 117, 142
silicon 138
sinus problems 73
sinusitis 49, 73–4
skin 35
skin brushing 78, 102, 119, 147–8
skin disorders 46, 72, 117–20, 130, 135
skipping meals 30, 55, 87, 95, 104
sleep 15, 77, 95, 135, 136
sleep-inducers 96
sleeping pills 96
slippery elm 122, 142–3
slow-release foods 37, 106, 116
small intestine 14, 19, 20–1, 51
smoking 24, 25, 48, 88, 101, 103, 108
snacks 56, 60, 65, 71, 88, 103, 106
soft drinks 113, 144
soup 59, 106, 113
sourdough 99, 134–5
soya 77, 140, 143
spelt 143
spicy foods 100, 122
spirulina 124
sprouts 59–60, 140
starch 51–6, 59, 70, 97, 101, 107, 113, 118
stomach 18, 20, 21–2
  acidity 22–3, 51–2
  inflamed 18

stomach cancer 22, 120, 133
stomach ulcer 18
stress 23, 29, 30, 37, 40–1, 45, 70, 75, 81, 88, 94, 101, 111–13, 118, 126, 127, 135, 144, 150
sugar 20, 21, 39, 46, 54, 64, 70–1, 79, 89, 100, 103, 110, 115, 118–19, 143–4
sulphur 70, 134, 138
supper 56, 96
supplements 56, 69, 102
suppositories 84
swimming 82, 84, 88
systemic lupus 23

tea 36, 57, 82, 88, 91, 113
teeth 20, 132
temperature 103, 110
tension, *see* stress
thirst 52
thyme 71, 72, 74, 77, 110, 144
tiredness 31, 51
tissue 39
toast 80
tomato 99, 101, 122
toxins 12, 20, 23, 38–9, 49
  overload 61
trace elements 40, 56, 85, 102, 118, 123, 127, 138
traveller's tummy 80
tuning 73

Udo's oil 82, 88, 102, 117, 119–20, 144
ulcer 15, 18, 23, 94, 120–2, 136
Umeboshi plum 77, 83, 144, 149
undigested food 22, 23, 31, 50, 97, 100
  protein 81, 83, 90, 97
uric acid 81
urinary problems 135
urine 20, 146–7

vaginitis 23
valerian 96, 115, 144
vegetable stock 56, 59–60, 85, 113
vegetables 34, 53–5, 59–60, 94, 97
  green leafy 71, 74
  raw 35, 55, 97, 122
vegetarian diet 52, 54
verbena/vervain 96, 145
villi 14, 134
viral disorders 108–11, 125, 130
vitamins 11, 19, 20, 21, 118
  supplements 69, 102, 138
  Vitamin A 126
  Vitamin B12 22
  Vitamin C 108, 136
volume of meal 31–2, 55, 77, 82, 83, 85, 87, 97, 102, 107, 110, 121, 123

walking 86, 88
water 35–6, 55, 56, 63, 76, 79, 82, 85–6, 113, 150
water therapy 79, 84
weight gain 31, 37
weight loss 63, 78
wheat 71, 74, 85, 134
wind 40, 49, 50–1, 55, 98, 100, 125, 133, 144, 145
work 42, 44, 58–60

yam, wild 112
yoga 73, 96
yoghurt 54, 55